BELLY BUSTING

BELLY BUSTING

FOR MEN

Nicole Senior & Veronica Cuskelly

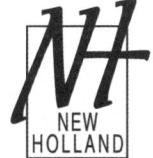

CONTENTS

INTRODUCTION	7
1. GET WITH THE PROGRAMME	8
2. MOVING TO BUST YOUR BELLY	30
3. MAN vs FOOD	46
4. CONQUER THE KITCHEN & SHRINK YOUR BELLY	72
Belly-busting Recipes	87
5. HOW TO LOVE FOOD & BUST YOUR BELLY	160
6. WAIST MATTERS	186
FURTHER INFORMATION	197
ACKNOWLEDGEMENTS	203
INDEX OF RECIPES	204

10 REASONS TO BUST YOUR BELLY

1. You'll look more attractive.

2. Your clothes will fit better.

3. Your lover will be able to wrap both arms around you.

4. You can go to the beach or pool without feeling embarrassed.

5. You'll have more energy to keep up with the younger crowd.

6. You'll perform better in bed.

7. You'll fit better behind the wheel.

8. Clipping your toenails will be so much easier.

9. You'll spend less on medical care and drugs (and more on hobbies, travel and other fun stuff).

10. Exercise, sport and any physical activity will be easier.

Over to you ...

INTRODUCTION

We wrote this book for you because we want you to feel good, look better, feel proud of yourself and get the most out of life.

We love the way you are logical and uncomplicated about food. We know you like to get straight down to business so we've put all the action in the front end of this book. The 'how-to' stuff is in Parts 1, 2 and 3 and the recipes are in Part 4: the 'why' stuff comes in the later sections. This is one owner's manual where you can get stuck in before you explore the many benefits of doing it and how it works.

We know you've got a lot on your plate, and sometimes it's not that good for you. We know you're not as clued-up on food and find the whole healthy eating thing a bit of a challenge. We know even thinking about your own health and wellbeing falls off your priority list, and we know you are bothered by your belly and would like to get rid of it. We believe in you and know that once you put your mind to something and have the right information, you are formidable.

Take our hands as we guide you through the belly-busting process. We promise we've made it easy and you will feel great for taking control of your body, your health and your life.

We know you can bust your belly and we're here to show you how. Ready ... set ... GO!

—Nicole Senior & Veronica Cuskelly

PART 1

GET WITH THE PROGRAMME

There's a US television show called *Overhaulin'* which takes a clapped-out old car ready for the scrapheap and does it up into something really special. Of course it takes months of hard work but it's totally worth it.

Take the same approach with your body and your lifestyle. It will take some effort and won't happen overnight but the results will be worth it

Think of this book as your overhaulin' toolkit. Right from page one, day one, we give you the how-to on what to eat and how much so you can bust your belly.

You get to choose how hard you want to go at 'overhaulin' right now.

Just as the road to success in anything is never straight, you can expect to have a few bumps in the road and maybe a breakdown or two on your belly busting journey. Hang in there and have faith in yourself—you are headed in the right direction. Here we go.

- 5 steps to bust your belly
- Choose your belly busting level
- TOP GEAR busting
- HIGH GEAR busting
- CRUISING
- How to stay on track

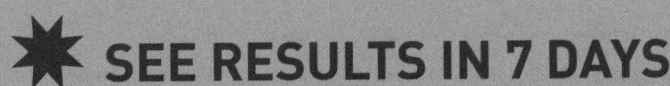 **SEE RESULTS IN 7 DAYS**

5 STEPS TO BUST YOUR BELLY

1. **Choose top-quality fuel.**
2. **Don't overfill your tank (if you do, go easy on food the next day).**
3. **Get your fuel mix right.**
4. **Put some miles on the clock.**
5. **Put your brain into gear (focus—think what you can eat, not what you can't).**

Choosing **top-quality fuel** simply means you give your body the fuel it needs to protect your health and improve your performance in every aspect of life. You get out what you put in, and you deserve the best.

We tell you straight—there's no sugar coating it—you need to **eat less** to bust your belly, but there are ways and means to do this without you needing to eat the leg of a chair (or the belly out of a low-flying duck).

We also give you ammunition to help you fight your way through eating in the wild of the modern food jungle, as well as in domestic captivity.

The **fuel mix** you put into your body is just as important as race fuel in a Formula One car. You need it to be balanced between the food groups and nutrients to give you the right mix of power and endurance, and it must be fuel that burns efficiently and cleanly (with no nasty residues).

Your body was **designed to move** and parking it indoors is a fast track to seizing up and becoming a wreck. You need to move regularly to keep your equipment in working order and give yourself the strength and fitness to cope with what life throws at you. You also need to move more to bust your belly.

Our belly busting programme explains what exercise actually works, how much you need to do and how you can make it happen in your daily life. Yes, I know you are busy working long hours/tied to your desk/no spare dates in your diary …

You can lead a horse to water … but you can't make him drink. I can give you the to-do and how-to lists but you need to make the **commitment** and **shift your mind into action**. If you don't, it's all just book-learning. What can help is focusing on the positive and setting realistic goals. A confident bloke is an unstoppable one.

Today your belly, tomorrow the world!

Wipe the slate clean

Hands up if you've been on a diet? Keep your hand up if you lost the weight and kept it off? Yep, that's typical: join the club. Chances are you've started diets full of good intentions. You may have done really well and been really strict with yourself for a week, maybe even two (some guys even manage a month). But then, real life kicked in. You started to feel hungry, unsatisfied and perhaps even pissed off that all your efforts were amounting to very little.

Where was the reward? You felt deprived, ripped off and maybe even a bit depressed. Then, just to vent your disappointment and frustration you might have gone on a bender, either with food or booze—or maybe both. Your way of saying, 'Stuff you, diet!' Any weight you lost came back, plus extra, and your confidence was chipped away each time this cycle was repeated. I'm asking you to let all that past stuff go, and don't get mad ... get back in control.

This is belly busting without the hocus-pocus, mumbo-jumbo, over-hyped pills and potions, airbrushed before and after photos or empty promises. There are no big bucks up front plus regular monthly payments, or special branded foods.

This is belly busting in the real world for real men. Gentleman, start your engines ...

CHOOSE YOUR BELLY-BUSTING LEVEL

NUMBER CRUNCH

Say an average man with a big belly needs around 11,000kJ (2627 calories) a day. If he only gets 3350kJ (800 calories) on a VLCD, he will get the remaining 7650kJ (1827 calories) from his fat stores. Theoretically, this represents a loss of 1.7kg a week—more if he uses energy for physical activity—and blokes typically lose between 1.5–2.5kg (3¼–5½lb) per week on a VLCD. If he can stick to it for a month, he could lose 6.7kg (14¾lb) : blokes typically lose 15–20kg (33–44lb) over 3 months.

Top gear busting

If you'd like to give yourself a major kick-start to busting your belly, you want quick results and you are fully committed and motivated, you can start with top gear using a Very Low Calorie Diet (VLCD) shakes. I recommend top gear for:

- men with bigger bellies
- men who are OK with not eating regular food for a while
- men with health issues like high blood pressure, high blood glucose, dodgy joints or sleep apnoea (snoring like a train)
- men who've been told by their doctor that they need to bust their belly
- men on a belly-busting deadline (for a significant event like a wedding).

High gear busting

If you'd prefer to eat regular healthy foods in controlled amounts, and bust your belly more gradually, you can follow our high gear programme.

Cruising

When you've achieved a belly size you're happy with, it's time for the cruising programme. Like when using the cruise control in your car, don't fall asleep at the wheel—you still need to keep your wits about you to keep active and eat the right food.

You can always change down a gear to have a breather. Change up again when you're ready.

THE TOP GEAR BUSTING PROGRAMME

To bust your belly you need to cut back on fuel and start to use up your reserves. The more fuel you cut back, the more belly reserves you'll use. An effective way to cut back without feeling like you're starving is to replace regular foods with specially designed diet shakes called Very Low Calorie Diets (VLCDs).

Quality VLCD products such as Optifast® and Slim&Save contain plenty of protein to conserve your muscle and essential vitamins and minerals so you don't go short. Crucially, they contain significantly fewer kilojoules than you would regularly eat; around 3350 kJ (800 calories) a day compared with 8000–10,000 kJ (2000–2388 calories). They also have protein bars and soups when you need a change from shakes.

You need to drink plenty of water and eat some non-starchy vegetables, such as carrots, broccoli, mushrooms or beans, each day.

You also shouldn't just stop the top gear programme suddenly, but gradually wean off the shakes and replace them with regular healthy food.

Of course you can't live like this forever—a month or two at most.

The pros and cons

Busting your belly in top gear will allow you to lead a busy life without having to think much about what to eat. This is a plus in the short term—however, you will still need to learn to feed yourself properly when you slip back into high gear and ease your way into cruising. You'll need to take your VLCD with you when you're away from home, and be prepared to forego regular food at social events. On the up side, it's not forever. It's a brave step towards a smaller belly and better health.

KILOJOULE OR CALORIE?

The kilojoule (kJ) is the modern unit for measuring energy contained in food. A calorie is the old unit, but many people don't like change (even though the kilojoule is the International System (SI) unit and was first proposed in 1977).

If you think of your body like a furnace, a food's kilojoule content is how much heat it creates when you digest and metabolise it. Unlike a furnace, however, your body stores excess kilojoules as fat—often in your belly. Restricting kilojoules causes your body to release stored energy and 'burn' fat to fuel your body's needs.

Ask your doctor or pharmacist for advice about VLCDs and check the website of the VLCD you choose for more detailed information and advice. For example: Optifast.com, Slimandsave.co.uk

Very Low Calorie Diets (VLCDs)

The effectiveness of Very Low Calorie Diets (VLCDs) is supported by many scientific studies. Doctors and dietitians have been recommending them for years when more rapid weight loss is required. They are not a fad diet. Don't be put off by the marketing hype of some brands: they really work. Big men have achieved amazing results in a pilot study led by dietitian Dr Penny Small in which they used Optifast® for a few months and then eased back into a low GI, moderate protein diet similar to high gear.

Won't I be really hungry?

Interestingly, radically cutting back on fuel using a VLCD does not increase hunger. In fact, the opposite usually happens and you feel less hungry. This is probably because the body goes into a state called ketosis whereby fat is being used for fuel rather than the usual sugars—and this dulls the hunger signals.

✸ Top gear how-to

- If you are taking any medication or are managing a chronic illness, check with your doctor before you start. Your medication may need adjusting.
- Start by using the shakes to replace all meals each day. This will achieve the most rapid belly busting.

During top gear, the only regular food you can eat are salads and low kilojoule vegetables such as broccoli, capsicum, carrot, celery, cucumber, fennel, green beans, lettuce, tomato, zucchini.

- The only food you can eat while on this top-gear phase is salads and low kilojoule vegetables. You can drink all the water, diet drinks and unsweetened black tea/coffee you like.
- Walk (or do other exercise) as much as you can to help your muscles stay strong while you're belly busting.
- Do this for as long as you are able. The bigger your belly, the longer you can stay on this intensive belly-busting phase—a month or two.
- If you have a social event you don't want to miss where

you can't avoid eating, have a modest meal and get back into top gear the next day. Expect your rate of belly-busting to slow for that week, and that you'll experience some rebound hunger.

Men's wisdom—my advice for other men
John, aged 49, accountant

What advice would I give to other men wanting to bust their belly?

- Decide for yourself if you are an important human being.
- If the answer is yes, set an appropriate but realistic goal and take expert advice on how to get there. Reading about maintaining a positive mental attitude is useful.
- Be prepared for some discomfort, both from exercise and changing eating habits—but know it's doing you heaps of good.
- Be proud of your goals and your achievements. This will feed back into points 1 and 2.

THE HIGH GEAR BUSTING PROGRAMME

SIZE	WAIST (CM)	WAIST (IN)
M	94–96	37–38
L	97–101	38–40
XL	102 cm+	40+

Note: these may not exactly match your clothing size measurements as these can vary considerably.

Choose your level

Because men of different sizes have varying food needs, we've designed three different levels within the high gear and cruising food plans: medium (M), large (L) and extra large (XL). Match yourself according to your waist size and follow the corresponding plan.

To make things easy, we've made the meals the same for men of all sizes—it's just the snacks and treats that are different.

Check your numbers

- If you're shorter than average, slip back a level because your body needs less food. For example, if your waist puts you in the XL zone but you're shorter than average, follow the plans for L.
- If you're over 60, slip back a level (from L to M, for example) because your body needs less overall food (sorry, but it's a fact!).
- If your weight is stuck on a plateau after following the plan for a while, slip back a level—you need to cut back on food to push through to a smaller belly.
- If you're very active, move up a level because you need more food. Or you could stay where you are and bust your belly faster (if you get too hungry, you can always move back up again).

Choose your food

There are DIY ideas as well as recipes in Part 4 (pages 72–159) to choose from. With eight different options for each meal, there are heaps of choices to keep things interesting week after week. But if you like sticking to the one breakfast or just a few lunches—go ahead. Want to eat your main meal at lunchtime? Go for it. Do whatever suits you.

You can relax about the nutritional balance and kilojoules too—we've worked it all out for you. All you need to do is choose, prepare, eat and enjoy!

Each day choose a breakfast, lunch, dinner, snacks and treat(s) according to your level.

Men's wisdom—the power of lower GI carbs
Geoff, aged 61, mining engineer

My life is a race from place to place and I spend a lot of time away from home. My belly has been gradually getting bigger for 10 years and then I got diabetes. Still, it took my first heart attack to get me to focus on my health. I got the fright of my life. It just made sense to take action. If I didn't change my lifestyle, I might die. I want to be around to see my grandkids grow up

I went about things in a logical and systematic way. I got all the information from my doctor, family doctor, dietitian and exercise specialist and went about re-organising my life. I got a lot of support from my wife too. Once I found out the facts, it was obvious where I'd been going wrong. I have changed my daily routine. I now exercise every day no matter where I am and think about what I eat a lot more.

I try to eat a bit of everything but I'm getting used to eating less. I don't skip meals any more—I make time for them and plan ahead for where I'll be. I also try to choose lower GI carbs when I can. I eat less rubbish in the car now too—I just don't buy it, and nibble on almonds or dried fruit instead. I drink considerably less than I used to: I just told my friends and colleagues I can't any more because of my diabetes.

It took me about four months, but then I felt great. I just feel better now in every way, and like I did 20 years ago. I only wish I'd worked it out sooner but you can't turn back the clock. I've lost 11cm off my waist and can now climb three flights of stairs in my office building. My diabetes has improved significantly. I've had to get rid of a whole bunch of 'fat' trousers but I'm glad. I've got a whole new lease on life and just feel happier.

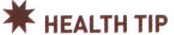
HEALTH TIP

Start your day with a tall glass of plain water (make it warm in winter). This will get your bowels moving and rehydrate you after sleep. Add a squeeze of lemon juice if you like.

Get with the Programme

8 BREAKFASTS

Choose any of these breakfasts to start your day well ... with quality food that tastes good and keeps you satisfied.

- 2/3 cup muesli (½ cup if toasted)
or
- Mix (page 88) *Raisin, cranberry and walnut grain-ola*
and
1 cup low-fat milk
1 large banana

- 2 slices wholegrain toast with margarine and Marmite or peanut butter
or
- 1 breakfast drink
or
- skim latte
1 large apple

- 4 wheat cereal biscuits
1 cup low-fat milk
2 tablespoons chopped mixed nuts (from supermarkets)
½ cup canned fruit pieces
or
- Cereal (page 89) *Bix, fruit and pecans*

- Melt (page 92) *Tomato, basil, bean and two cheeses*

- ¾ cup porridge oats made with 1 cup low-fat milk
2 tablespoons raisins or sultanas
or
- Porridge (page 90) *Oats with honey and rhubarb*

- 2 cups (90g) of high-fibre breakfast cereal (eg wholewheat flakes & sultanas)
1 cup low-fat milk
½ cup canned peach slices, drained

Weekend special

- 2 eggs on 2 slices wholemeal/grain toast with margarine and sautéed tomatoes and mushrooms in a little oil
or
- Fry (page 91) *Bacon 'n' egg brekkie*
2/3 cup 100% fruit juice

- Mushrooms (page 95) *Sherry and smoked paprika mushrooms*

✳ Breakfast tips

- Use a measuring cup when serving your cereal to ensure the right amount—at least at first. After that you can probably eyeball it (but watch out for portion creep or changing your bowl size).
- Look for low-GI bread for your toast and lower GI breakfast cereals. Low-GI breads are dense, grainy breads containing soy, seeds, oats and/or barley. As well as muesli and porridge, lower GI cereals tend to be high in bran or based on wholewheat. Check the label for the GI symbol, or check the database at www.glycemicindex.com. Enter the word 'cereal' and search for those less than GI 60.
- Top up the juice with water to fill your glass.

Caffeine lovers

Instant coffee or tea with a little low-fat milk is OK any time of the day. To avoid caffeine overload, limit espresso or percolated coffee to no more than three (regular-sized) cups a day. Try using a sweetener instead of sugar if you have more than two or three cups a day. I reckon brands made with sucralose or stevia taste the best, but taste them and decide yourself. Over time it's a good idea to wean yourself off sweetness in your cuppa altogether. A sweet tooth gets more demanding the more you indulge it.

Break-the-fast
Skipping breakfast is a bad idea. Get up earlier if you need to, or eat breakfast at work. Just eat it.

CHOOSING A HIGH-FIBRE CEREAL

Don't bamboozle yourself with the numbers on the side of the box. Look for the words 'high fibre' on the front and at least 10g/100g (10%) fibre content on the nutrition panel.

NUMBER CRUNCH

The breakfasts opposite are all around 2000 kJ (478 calories). Use this as a guide to help you put together your own ideas. You'll find that all our 'Breakfasts of champions' (page 88) and 'On-toast specials' (page 93) recipes are around this target.

Get with the Programme

8 LUNCHES

- 1 small wholemeal pita bread
  ½ cup hummus
  1 small tomato
  1 large orange (or other fruit)

- Wrap (page 99) *Egg, dukkah, mayonnaise and rocket*

- 2 thick slices of grain bread with margarine
  2 slices lite light ham or beef
  salad (eg, baby spinach, tomato)
  1 boiled egg
  1 large pear (or other fruit)

- Roll (page 98) *Mustard and horseradish beef salad*

- Salmon (page 96) *Salmon with lemon dill yoghurt*
  1 large grain roll with margarine

- 1 small can salmon or tuna (in water)
  salad (eg, lettuce, grated carrot, cucumber)
  1 large apple (or other fruit)

- 1 mixed grain muffin, split & and toasted
  ½ cup salt-reduced baked beans (a small can), warmed
  2 individual slices light cheese (melt under the grill)
  1 cup baby spinach leaves
  1 large banana

When you have a bit more time
- Noodles (page 100) *Tuna, sweet Soy, lemon ginger dressing*

✹ Lunch tips

- Fit in as much salad or cooked vegetables as you can because they do you good and fill you up without filling you out.
- Hardboil three or four eggs at the beginning of the week and keep them in the fridge to pack in your lunch box.
- Limit margarine to 1 teaspoon per slice of bread.
- You can swap fresh fruit for canned fruit.
- One large fruit can be swapped for two or three small ones (whatever fits in one hand).
- Baby spinach leaves are packed with nutrition and are ultra-convenient. Add them to salads, sandwiches or use as a bed for serving things on toast.

Men better at resisting food

US research using brain imaging has shown men are better than women at resisting tempting food treats and more able to switch off thoughts of food. The men in the study experienced less hunger and food cravings after going without food for a day and the area of the brain involved with emotion was less active in men than women. Women also have more body image anxiety as well as hormones to contend with.

NUMBER CRUNCH

The lunches opposite are all around 2000kJ (478 calories). Use this as a guide to help you put together your own ideas. You'll find all our 'DIY lunch' and 'On-toast specials' recipes are around this target (see pages 93–103).

Get with the Programme 21

NUMBER CRUNCH

The dinners opposite are all around 3000kJ (717 calories). Use this as a guide to help you put together your own ideas. You'll find our all-in-one main meal recipes are around this target, and the meal component recipes (eg roast meat and a salad) add up to meet it.

✷ Dinner tips

- You can swap different protein foods if you like—for example, switch chicken for veal or pork (as long as it's lean).
- You can swap the 200g (7oz) meat for 200g hard tofu or tempeh..
- Use whatever vegetable you like just make sure you have at least three different types (ideally different colours).
- The best way to cook vegetables is to steam, microwave or stir-fry to preserve their goodness.
- You can buy all kinds of stir-fry and simmer sauces in jars. Look for 'light' or 'reduced salt' options in flavours that you like.

What is ...

Tofu (bean curd) and tempeh are made from soy beans and are rich in protein. Soy bean milk is set into a smooth texture with calcium or magnesium salt (nigari) to make tofu. Tempeh is fermented soybean cake made from whole soy beans. You can use sliced or cubed hard tofu (not soft) or tempeh in place of meat in stir-fries. You can usually find them near the yoghurts in the supermarket chiller sold in 500g (1lb 2oz) slabs.

8 DINNERS

- 200g (7oz) lean chicken or beef strips
  1½–2 cups vegetables for stir-frying
  ¼ cup Asian style stir-fry sauce
  40g (1½oz) quick noodles (½ packet)
  or
- Stir-fry (page 134) *Pork, pepper and ginger*
  1 palmful unsalted cashews (30g/1oz)

- 200g (7oz) (raw weight) lean chicken
  1½–2 cups mixed vegetables
  ¼ jar (120g/4oz) light sauce for chicken
  ½ cup cooked brown rice
  or
- Curry (page 136) *Thai-style chicken*

- Meatloaf (page 122) *Beef and lentil*
  1 cup green peas

- 200g (7oz) lean pork steak, grilled
  green beans/broccoli (at least 1 cup)
  Spuds (page 126) *Creamy chive, bacon & pinenut*

- 2 white fish fillets (300g/10½oz)
  or
- 1 salmon steak/cutlet (150g/5oz), grilled or pan fried
  1 large cob corn (or 2 small) with 1 teaspoon margarine
  Tossed (page 125) *Mixed vegetable salad*

- Chilli (page 131) *Beef and bean chilli*
  side salad (eg, lettuce, pepper strips, cucumber and tomato)

When you've got some time ...
- Chicken (page 108) *Spiced Moroccan and lemon*
  Couscous (page 110) *Cumin potatoes, carrot and bean*

- Spag-bol (page 138) *Spaghetti and meat sauce*
  side salad

NOTE: All meat, fish and poultry weights are raw weights

SAFE SNACKS

- M men choose two snacks—one snack from Group A and one from B.
- L and XL men choose three snacks—one snack from Group A, one from B, plus an extra snack from either Group A or C.
- Eat these between meals, or add them to your meals.

Group A—choose 1 a day

These dairy snacks are around 600kJ (143 calories)—check the labels of other dairy snacks you find for other suitable options:

- medium glass of low-fat milk (1 small carton/300ml/10fl oz)
- breakfast drink (1 cup)
- large skim hot chocolate or skim latte
- small light flavoured milk or skim milkshake (about 1 cup)
- 1 tub low-fat yoghurt (200g/7oz)
- small skim fruit smoothie (about 1 cup)

Group B—choose 1 a day

These fruit snacks are around 300kJ (72 calories)—you can vary the fruits you choose:

- 1 large apple
- 1 banana
- 1 large pear
- 1 handful of grapes (about 20)
- ½ large can (200g/7oz) of fruit
- small handful of dried fruit (eg, 6 apricot halves or 2 tablespoons sultanas)

Group C

These snacks contain around 600kJ (143 calories):

- small palmful (30g/1oz) of unsalted nuts (whatever you like)
- 2 boiled eggs
- 220g (8oz) can baked beans (reduced salt)
- 1 plain oat-based muesli bar (no chocolate or coatings)
- 1 thick (toast-sized) slice mixed grain and seed bread with scrape of margarine or peanut butter

✸ Snack tips

- Dairy foods like milk and yoghurt are packed with goodness and keep you satisfied because of their protein content and low GI. You do need to keep them cold; transport them in an insulated bag with an ice brick.
- Many products nowadays are sold in large sized portions, such as light flavoured milk in 600ml (1pt) bottles or cartons. If need be, drink half and save the rest for the following day (provided you can keep it in the fridge). Or drink it all and forego a snack later in the day.
- Don't forget fruits that need to be cut up. Slices of delicious melons, pineapple and mangoes can be packed up in a sealed container to go. It saves time if you cut up the lot and keep it in a sealed container in your fridge, then dish it out as required.
- You can put smaller fruits like cherries, berries, plums and apricots into a container to go so they stay in good shape.

✸ And some tips about treats

- Belly busting doesn't have to mean banning all treats, just eating them less often and in small amounts. You have to have some room in your eating plan to socialise or partake in family fun food.
- You'll notice these are all modest portion sizes. If you can't stop eating them, then don't start—have an extra snack instead (see opposite). However, in the long run, you'll have to learn how to be around fattening food and not eat it (or eat very little).
- You can forego treats on some days—save them up to have a larger serve on another day, such as a weekend day.

TREATS

- M & L men choose one treat from either Group A or B.
- XL men choose two treats from either Group A or B, or one from Group C.

A treat from either Group A or B is around 300kJ (72 calories).
If you want to add your own options to this list, Group C treats (see opposite page) are around 600kJ (143 calories).

Group A

- ½ glass (100ml/2¾fl oz) wine

- ¾ cup popcorn
  or
  1 mini-pack potato crisps (25g/¾oz)

- 1 nip (30ml/1fl oz) spirits, plus diet mixer if you like

- 285ml (10fl oz) beer (twist-top)
  or
  450ml (14½fl oz) light (2% alcohol) beer

- 1 tub 'diet' chocolate mousse
  or
  'diet' crème caramel

Group B

- 2 small plain biscuits
  or
  1 rich biscuit (eg, chocolate-coated or cream-filled)

- 3 small squares chocolate
  or
  15 small candy-coated chocolates
  or
  6 chocolate-coated peanuts

- 1 ice block (eg, fruit flavoured) on a stick

- 1 short licorice stick (12cm/4¾in)
  or
  4 marshmallows
  or
  5 soft jelly lollies

- 1 small scoop low-fat ice cream
  or
  lower kilojoule (calorie) ice cream on a stick

Group C
Two treats worth of treat (two treats in one):

- 375ml (12fl oz) regular beer
- 1 small glass (200ml/7fl oz) wine
- double-nip of spirits (with 'diet' mixers only)
- 1 small slice fruit pie (eg, apple), 9cm (4in) wide at the crust edge
- 1 fruit bun (eg, hot cross bun)
- 1 muesli bar (30–40g/1–1½oz size)
- 1 small bag potato crisps (50g/1¾oz)
- 1 small nut bar
- 1 mini chocolate-coated ice cream
- 1 small tub dairy dessert (eg, chocolate custard)
- 1 tub rice pudding snack
- Ice (page 150: *Mango and apple granita*
- Sundae (page 143): *Mulled cherry and almond*

THE CRUISING PROGRAMME

When you're happy with the size of your belly, it's time to get into 'cruise' mode. How does this differ to high gear, you ask? Er, well, here's the thing. It doesn't. Allow me to explain …

To maintain your smaller belly high gear = cruising

If you're now a shadow of your former self and can see your toes again, your energy needs have actually reduced because there is less of you—and there are less hungry fat cells to feed. To think that you still have to watch the quantity of food you eat might seem cruel, but it's a metabolic fact. If you let it all go now, your belly will come straight back and this is physically and psychologically bad.

This means that high gear is what you need to do on a more permanent basis to maintain your smaller belly. To keep your belly small, high gear becomes cruising. Think of it as a road map—you can stray off the beaten track if you like, but you need to find your way back quickly to prevent getting totally lost and frustrated.

Remember, if your belly busting has stopped on high gear and you still want to keep shrinking your belly, you need to slip back a size. For example, slip back from L to M.

If you're a smaller man already following M and would like to shrink your belly further, remove a snack from Group B (page 24) and/or your treat (pages 26–27).

GETTING BACK ON TRACK

Life is busy and eating well is challenging. You need to expect some periods of your life to be more challenging to cruise than others. If evasive action is needed to avoid a crash, act early and decisively. Keep a sharp eye on the road to monitor the conditions to pre-empt problems.

> Failing to factor in the need to eat less after a diet than before is the reason many men experience weight rebound.

✹ Cruising tips

- If you overeat, eat less later on in the day or the next day and ramp up your exercise time or intensity.
- Keep track of your weight and waist size once a fortnight (or once a month if you're holding steady).
- If you have a major weight or waist blow out, get back into top gear to repair the damage. Don't do this too often — gaining and losing large amounts of weight repeatedly (weight cycling, or yo-yo dieting) is bad for your health.
- If you fall off the belly-busting wagon. Just accept what has happened and know you have the ability to get back on board. Remember, in the scheme of your whole life, this is small backward step. Like the stockmarket, keep your eye on the general (downward) trend of the size of your belly rather than the small fluctuations.

What is ... metabolism?

The term metabolism (or metabolic rate) refers to the amount of energy the body uses each day — like a daily energy budget — and is measured as kilojoules per day.

Metabolism consists of three basic components: Basal Metabolic Rate (BMR); thermogenesis, and physical activity. There are ways you can boost your spending on all three fronts.

Basal Metabolic Rate is the energy you spend to keep your heart beating, your brain and nervous system firing, your muscles fed and your liver and kidneys working. Your BMR is primarily related to your lean body mass, so developing and maintaining muscle is a great way to spend more energy (even when you're sitting still!).

Thermogenesis is the energy you spend to digest and metabolise your food. Starving yourself lowers your energy budget as well as having the obvious negative physical and psychological consequences. Eat regular meals and enough protein as you need more energy to help with belly busting.

METABOLISM MYTHS

Some people say repeatedly losing and gaining weight wrecks (permanently lowers) your metabolism, but this is incorrect. Your metabolism (metabolic rate, or fuel-burning rate) is based on the sum of your lean body mass, how much you eat and how much you exercise.

Weight loss lowers your metabolic rate and weight gain increases it. Eating more increases your metabolic rate and eating less decreases it. Doing more exercise increases metabolic rate and doing less decreases it.

PART 2

MOVING TO BUST YOUR BELLY

Physical activity is perhaps the most obvious way to increase your metabolism, and the more you do the more energy you'll spend. You can start today and the effects are immediate. If you do some high-intensity exercise, you will continue to spend energy for hours after you stop exercising.

You've gotta move. We were built to move. End of story. We help you to understand why you need to move, the best moves to do and how to fit more of them into your life.

- Why movement is the best medicine
- What's the difference between activity and exercise?
- How much and how often?
- New belly-busting exercise on the block
- What about strength training?
- The best exercise to bust your belly
- Tips and tricks
- Resistance exercises
- A beginner's exercise programme

'I'm going for a walk to clear the cobwebs' is a saying that correctly sums up the benefits of movement for both body and mind. Walking to 'clear the head' describes the benefits for both thinking and mood.

WHY MOVEMENT IS THE BEST MEDICINE

Being sedentary places you at nearly twice the risk of developing heart disease than an active man.

If I told you that exercise was the best preventive medicine you could take, you probably wouldn't believe me. But it's true. If the benefits of exercise could be bundled into a pill and sold, it would be the most wildly profitable medicine of the modern age. But of course you can't take exercise in a pill.

Exercise helps to prevent over 20 diseases that blight men's lives (usually when they're just starting to relax and enjoy the fruits of their labours), including obesity, high blood pressure, diabetes, heart disease, stroke, some cancers, osteoporosis and depression, just to name a few. It also makes you feel better both physically and mentally.

'When I was a boy I had to walk 10 miles in bare feet to get to school' is a typical grandad story that is subject of many a family joke but it actually speaks volumes of how our level of physical activity has plummeted over time.

The human body was built to move, yet we have done our level best to engineer movement out of our lives. Cars, sedentary jobs, technology and the quest for convenience have all made it easier to do very little. If you want to be active, you usually have to plan to make it happen. Remember, your body was designed for hunting food and defending the family from wild animals—it's crying out for exercise. More aggro used on the punching bag and pounding the pavement means less aggro left directed towards yourself and others.

Apart from not smoking, being physically active is the most powerful step you can take for better health.

Being physically active reduces the risk of erectile dysfunction (impotence).

Exercise assists the imperfect man

It's a no-brainer that you'll be healthiest if you eat well, don't smoke, drink alcohol in moderation, have a flat belly and exercise. However, even if you smoke and/or have a big belly, exercise helps to minimise the damage. You can be 'fit and fat' and even if you haven't quit the fags you'll be better off if you exercise. Even without losing weight, exercise provides heaps of health benefits, but exercising while losing weight helps you burn more fat (bust your belly) while keeping your muscles intact.

Men's wisdom
Paul, aged 44, IT manager
I sit on my bum every day in front of a computer and rarely need to leave my desk. I always feel tired and rarely see my friends because I just don't have the energy after work. Of course I know I should be exercising more, but I found it difficult to fit it in. My doctor read me the riot act. I now do a weekly exercise plan at the beginning of each week to fit in what I can with the rest of my commitments. I also take the stairs in my building and get off the bus one stop early and walk home. I now walk in my lunch break a few times a week and I'm now working up to jogging with some workmates. I've lost 10kg [22lb] so far and my cholesterol has come down. I was a bit negative at first—I didn't think I was able to do enough to make any difference, but I have made a difference. I've changed my attitude and my wife is really pleased too.

Walking or cycling for more than 30 minutes a day reduces the risk of prostate cancer.

WHAT'S THE DIFFERENCE BETWEEN PHYSICAL ACTIVITY AND EXERCISE?
Like Paul, you might think unless you huff and puff and sweat like a maniac there's no point in doing anything active. You'd be wrong. The scientific evidence is convincing that any movement is beneficial: doing something is absolutely better than doing nothing. In fact, the most benefit can be gained from a couch potato who decides to get up and walk around a bit.

Physical activity is any body movement you do that uses

YOU'RE NEVER TOO OLD TO START
It doesn't matter whether you're 30, 40, 50, 60 or 70, increasing physical activity will benefit you by reducing your risk of disease and keeping your body and mind in better working order.

The potential benefits from becoming physically active are greatest in those who are currently doing nothing (sedentary).

Moving to Bust Your Belly 33

energy. Getting up off the couch and going outside to get the mail is physical activity.

Exercise is planned physical activity you do for fun (like sport) or for health and fitness (like power walking or jogging).

Incidental physical activity is movement you do as part of your daily life, like walking to the bus stop or washing the car.

MODERATE OR VIGOROUS?
Moderate-intensity physical activity

This is movement that moderately and noticeably increases your depth of breathing and breathing rate, while still allowing you to comfortably talk (eg, cycling for pleasure or brisk walking). For example:

- aquarobics (water aerobics)
- brisk walking
- cycling
- swimming
- surfing and body boarding (which is higher intensity for beginners who need to work harder)
- golf (walking between holes—no buggies please!)
- dancing
- active gardening and/or yard work.

There's a more specific scale used to measure how hard you're working during exercise. Ratings of Perceived Exertion (RPE) are simple ways of assessing your exercise intensity. This scale (right) of zero to 10 is called the OMNI Scale of Perceived Exertion. Moderate is 5–6 and Vigorous is 7–8.
Source: Robert J Robertson, *Validation of the Adult OMNI Scale of Perceived Exertion for Walking/Running Exercise, Medicine and Science in Sports & Exercise* (2004).

0	Extremely easy	
1		
2	Easy	
3		
4	Somewhat easy	
5		
6	Somewhat hard	MODERATE
7		
8	Hard	VIGOROUS
9		
10	Extremely hard	

Vigorous-intensity physical activity

This is movement at a higher intensity which, depending on your fitness level, may cause sweating and puffing. For example:

- running
- netball or basketball
- soccer
- rugby or touch rugby
- football
- tennis or squash
- uphill walking
- aerobics
- circuit training
- rowing
- stair climbing
- gym circuit classes.

How much and how often?

On top of any incidental activity you accumulate in your day:

- aim for a minimum of 30 minutes of moderate-intensity aerobic exercise (such as brisk walking) on five days each week OR vigorous-intensity exercise for a minimum of 20 minutes three days each week (such as jogging)
- a combination of moderate and vigorous exercise can be used to meet the guidelines
- strength training two days a week using the major muscle groups with a load that allows eight to 12 repetitions until you feel muscle fatigue.

Source: American College of Sports Medicine and the American Heart Association

See movement as an opportunity not an inconvenience.

WHAT IS...
Aerobic exercise is fat-burning exercise needing oxygen which makes your heart beat faster and your lungs breathe harder.

SAVE TIME, GO HARDER
Aim for at least 150 minutes per week of moderate-intensity physical activity (such as brisk walking). If you have little time, you can reduce this time to 60 minutes a week by doing vigorous exercise (such as jogging).

Remember these are a minimum. The more exercise you do, the more benefits you'll get. To bust your belly, more or longer sessions are needed. In fact, cancer prevention experts say you should be doing at least 60 minutes of moderate-intensity exercise a day to reduce your risk.

Moving to Bust Your Belly

ACTIVE TRANSPORT

If you struggle to commit to a sporting team or attend a gym, then join the masses who are embracing active transport, either on foot or on a bike.

This is the ultimate activity with purpose: you're simply using your body power to get where you need to go. Active commuting is a passport to health (and cleaner air), but even if this is not possible for you every day, walk or cycle as much as you can.

Active commuting is the perfect energising start to the day and the perfect after-work therapy that allows you to perform well at work and be a nicer guy at home.

Active commuting reduces the risk of developing cardiovascular disease. If you need to look shmick at work, take a change of clothes (or keep clothes at work).

Check with your doctor

If you've got any health issues then please talk to your doctor before you do any vigorous exercise. Check with your doctor if ...

- you have a heart condition and can only do physical activity recommended by a doctor
- you feel pain in the chest when you do physical activity or exercise
- you have had chest pain in the last month, even when you weren't doing physical activity
- you lose your balance because of dizziness or ever lose consciousness
- you have bone or joint problems that could be made worse by a change in your physical activity
- you are currently prescribed medication for high blood pressure.

—American College of Sports Medicine

> **✷ BREAK IT DOWN**
>
> If the thought of putting aside 30 minutes a day is daunting, don't panic. Studies have shown you can improve your fitness by breaking it down into shorter bouts over the day. This means if you can't spare 30 minutes to take a walk, you can do two lots of 15 minutes or three lots of 10 minutes.

Lunchtime workouts

Many men struggle to fit in exercise before and after work because of long commutes or work hours. Try lunchtime activity, whether at the local gym or park. Create a social aspect by enlisting workmates to join you—it's always harder to pike out if you know your mates are counting on you.

Men's wisdom

Frank, aged 52, university lecturer (and successful belly buster)
When I was younger I played football and it kept me fit and trim. When that ended I started running with a running club. But when injuries stopped me I found that it was all too easy to stop training completely: why bother, what for, I'll never get back to where I was ... Of course, the outcome was a steady increase in weight. I reckon with middle age, kids, etc, it is just so easy to drift into excess weight, reduced cardio fitness and muscle loss. So I'm a great believer in having a challenge to keep you going. Having a good reason to train hard is important and competitive clubs of one sort or another are a good source of motivation. So at present I'm a member of a cycling club which races two or three times per month and this provides me with an incentive to do 90 to 125 miles per week training plus being careful (but not crazy) with what I eat. What's really motivating is that every four pounds I lose saves me six grand. How so? A road bike that is about four pounds lighter than my current one costs £6000 more, so that each couple of pounds I lose I reckon is like saving £3000!

NEW BELLY-BUSTING EXERCISE ON THE

But we don't have showers ...
Don't let the absence of showers at your work prevent you from exercising. Make it work, no excuses. A towel and a good deodorant are all you need to freshen up.

GET YOURSELF A PEDOMETER
This little gadget you wear on your belt counts how many steps you take each day. Establish your usual number (baseline) and then set small increases week by week. A good target is 10,000 steps a day—but you may want to start with 7500.

Moving to Bust Your Belly

BLOCK: INTERVAL TRAINING

You've probably done interval training without calling it that. Interval training is alternating between higher intensity exercise and lower intensity exercise (or recovery periods). It's about going hard, then going easy, and repeating this. For example, doing running intervals within your brisk walking session. If you're not up to running, then it could be alternating between slow and fast walking (even on a treadmill). If you cycle, this is alternating between cruising and sprinting. It even works in swimming.

What's good about Interval training?
- Excellent for burning fat.
- Great for boosting fitness.
- Reduces the time needed to burn the same amount of energy (saves exercise time).

How to do interval training

Start off slow and gradually increase the challenge level. If you have any health problems, talk to your doctor to get the OK to do high-intensity exercise.

- Do one or two interval training sessions per week.
- If you're starting at a low intensity (such as slow walking), gradually increase the pace of both the lower and higher intensity exercise.
- Include one or two four-minute hard intervals at first, and gradually increase to four four-minute intervals with three minutes recovery in between.

Whatever exercise you do, it's good to warm up and cool down for around five minutes before and after. It's also a good idea to do some gentle stretches of the muscles you use after an exercise session.

STRENGTH TRAINING

Doing some strength training, also known as resistance exercise, improves muscular size, strength and endurance. Resistance exercise is a method of conditioning muscles, joints and bones that involves the progressive use of resistance to increase your ability to exert force. It challenges your muscles by overloading them so they get stronger. Lifting weights is an example, and so is using resistance bands or using your body weight such as when doing a push-up. Resistance training does not mean body building, which is a separate exercise category with little relevance to the everyday bloke.

What is resistance exercise?
- Free weights (such as dumbbells)
- Weight machines
- Rowing machine
- Push ups
- Sit ups
- Jumps
- Chin ups
- Tricep dips
- Lunges and squats
- (Elastic) resistance bands
- Fitness ball
- Pilates

Resistance exercise is good because it:
- helps burn fat
- strengthens muscles
- strengthens bones
- increases metabolic rate
- improves metabolic fitness (eg, improves blood pressure, insulin and glucose levels, etc)
- improves mood
- helps back pain.

How to start

If you've not done resistance exercise before, start off slowly and build up the length of the session and the number of sessions per week. If you're using weights, make sure you learn the correct technique: start with a light weight before increasing the weight. Increase the weight as your strength increases—the weight should have your muscle feeling fatigued at the end of a set (not halfway through). It's a good idea to get expert help from a trainer or exercise physiologist at first so you know you're doing the exercises correctly.

Because you're working your muscles until they tire, you need to leave at least a day between sessions to give them a chance to recover. Expect some soreness in the muscles you used in the two days following resistance training, particularly when you first start. This is a normal part of muscle recovery and even has a name: Delayed Onset Muscle Soreness (DOMS).

- Do 8 to 10 different exercises working on different muscle groups (eg, front of legs, calves, chest, back, front and back of arms). Exercise large muscle groups such as your glutes (the muscles in your buttocks) and chest before smaller muscle groups like your calves and biceps.
- Start with one set of 10 to 15 repetitions ('reps') and build up to three sets of 8 to 12 reps with a heavier load, taking one to two minutes rest between each set.
- Build up to two or three sessions a week.
- Don't hold your breath—breathe out during exertion.

✸ Exercising tips

- Keep a bag of exercise clothes and shoes at work or in your car so you're ready for action.
- If you're finding it hard to start up in the mornings, lay out your exercise clothes ready for the mornings.
- Listen to music, podcasts or your favourite radio station in your headphones to make walking or jogging more enjoyable.
- Arrange regular walking with family or friends.
- Choose activities you enjoy doing, and keep things varied to maintain your interest.
- Wear comfortable clothing and footwear. If you're overheating or getting blisters on your feet, you'll be less likely to continue.
- Drink plenty of water before, during and after exercise to stay well hydrated.

The best belly-busting exercise

The best exercise is exercise you can do regularly and like enough to keep doing it.

You can see an exercise physiologist for a tailored programme to meet your specific goals, but in the long term you just need to do more than you're doing now—and make it part of your life. There's little point starting exercise for your belly-busting programme and then abandoning it once you've lost a few inches: that's a fast track to having a big belly again.

Men's wisdom
David, 52, self-employed
David had just recovered from a heart attack that gave him the fright of his life. David was highly motivated to get his health back on track and made the necessary changes to his diet. But despite understanding the importance of exercise, he just couldn't make it happen—there were always competing priorities for his time. He liked the idea of walking along the beach but hated going on his own. His wife Wendy agreed to start walking with him. David and Wendy walk most mornings and it has now become an enjoyable part of their day. David found having the company and support of his wife was important in starting this new healthy habit. Both David and Wendy have lost inches around their bellies. As David works long hours, they both really enjoy the opportunity to talk while on their walk as well.

RESISTANCE EXERCISES
The following exercises can be done at the gym or at home with resistance bands or dumbbells. If you're not ready to purchase your own equipment, you can use large milk or detergent bottles filled with water or sand. Of course, you can substitute similar activities for these ones if you prefer, or use the weights machines if you are attending a gym. Remember to wear enclosed shoes to protect your feet. All resistance exercise needs to be slow, smooth and controlled. Focus your mind on the muscle group you are using.

Exercise	How to	How to make it harder
Squats	Stand with feet shoulder width apart and squat down as far as you can go, pushing your hips back and bending your knees. Keep your weight on your heels and don't let your knees go past your toes. Pause, then slowly push yourself back to the starting position.	*Use weights:* Extend hands out front and hold weights in your hands while arms are extended.
Seated row	*Use weights:* Sit or stand with your back straight and start with arms fully extended. Slowly pull hand weights towards your chest, bringing your elbows to your sides and squeezing your shoulder blades together while keeping your neck and shoulders relaxed. Push the weights back out again.	Increase weight.
Push-ups	Kneel on the floor and lean forward to support your weight with your arms, placing your hands directly under your shoulders. Keeping your arms straight and ensuring your hands are a shoulder-width apart, slowly lower your body to the floor, ensuring you keep your back straight and taking care not to lock your elbows.	Move from balancing on knees to toes. *Use weights:* Carry a weight on your back (eg, placed in a backpack or even a small child if they can lie still!).

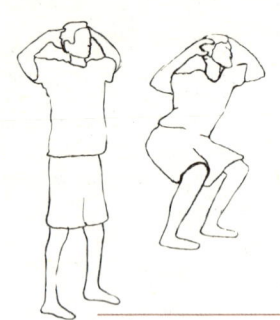

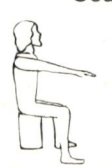

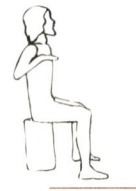

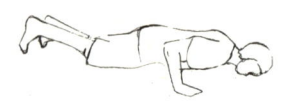

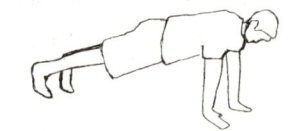

Moving to Bust Your Belly

Exercise	Instructions	Progression
Overhead press	*Use weights:* Stand up straight with your arms bent, hands at shoulder level elbows close to your ribs. Straighten arms upwards, pushing weights up and above your head. Slowly bend your elbows and lower the weights back down to starting position.	Increase weight.
Bicep curls 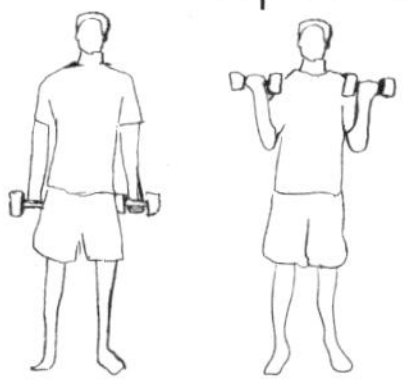	*Use weights:* With arms by your sides, weights in palms facing forward, bend each elbow to lift weight towards the shoulder and lower again.	Increase weight.
Tricep dips	Hold on to the edge of a bench, step or chair. Place feet flat on the floor with knees bent. With your weight towards your body, bend your elbows to raise and lower your body weight.	Extend your legs and keep feet on the floor, further away from your body. Place feet on another chair the same height as the one supporting your arms.
Heel raises	Stand with your feet a few inches apart on the edge of a step. Slowly rise onto the ball of your foot and lower again.	Move from standing on two feet to one foot. *Use weights:* Hold weights in your hands.
Abdominal crunches 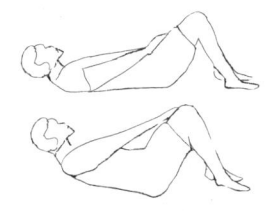	Lie on the floor with knees bent and hands on your thighs. Focusing on the abdominal muscles, exhale and lift the upper body off the ground, sliding your hands up to touch your knees, and lower again.	Place hands behind your head. *Use weights:* Hold weights in your hands, folded across your chest.

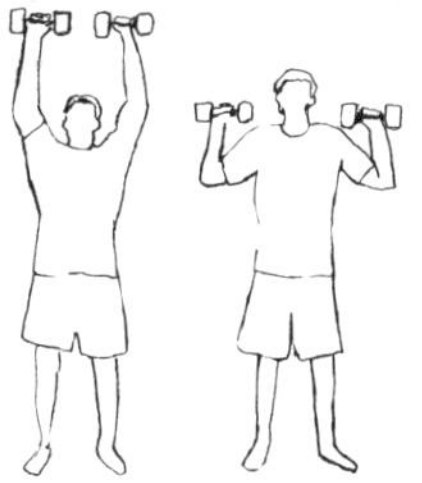

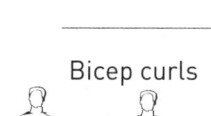

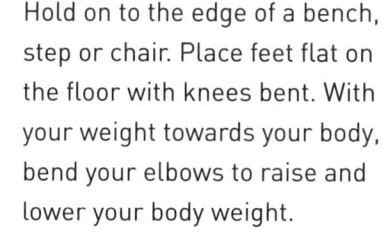

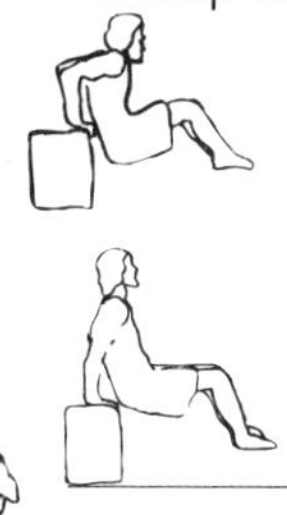

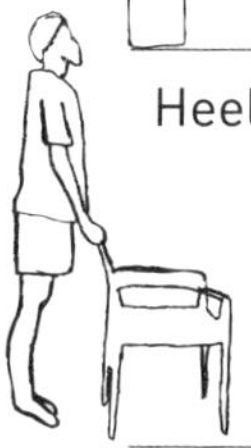

Moving to Bust Your Belly

A BEGINNER'S 8-WEEK EXERCISE PROGRAMME

This programme is designed for men who don't do much exercise and need an introduction to better fitness and a more active life.

Week	Mon	Tues	Wed
1	20-minute walk	Resistance training (1 set x 10 reps)	20-minute walk
2	30-minute walk	Resistance training (1 x 15)	30-minute walk
3	30-minute interval walk	15-minute walk Resistance training (2 x 15)	30-minute walk
4	20-minute walk Resistance training (2 x 15)	40-minute interval walk	20-minute walk Resistance training (2 x 15)
5	20-minute walk Resistance training (3 x 15)	45-minute interval walk	20-minute walk Resistance training (3 x 15)
6	25-minute walk Resistance training (3 x 12)	45-minute interval walk/jog	25-minute walk Resistance training (3 x 12)
7	30-minute walk Resistance training (3 x 12)	45-minute interval walk/jog	30-minute walk Resistance training (3 x 12)
8	30- min interval walk Resistance training (3 x 12)	50-minute interval walk/jog	30-minute interval walk Resistance training (3 x 12)

Moving to Bust Your Belly

Thurs	Fri	Sat	Sun
20-minute walk	Resistance training (1 x 12)	30-minute walk	Mow the lawn
30-minute walk	Resistance training (2 x 15)	30-minute walk	Game of golf
30-minute walk	15-minute walk Resistance training (2s x 15)	30-minute interval walk	Football with friends
40-minute interval walk	20-minute walk Resistance training (3 x 15)	40-minute interval walk	Bushwalk
45-minute interval walk	20-minute walk Resistance training (3 x 12)	45-minute interval walk	Mow the lawn
45-minute interval walk/jog	25-minute walk Resistance training (3 x 12)	45-minute interval walk/jog	Game of golf
45-minute interval walk/jog	30-minute walk Resistance training (3 x 12)	45-minute interval walk/jog	Football with friends
50-minute interval walk/jog	30-minute interval walk Resistance training (3 x 12)	50-minute interval walk/jog	Family cricket game

Moving to Bust Your Belly

PART 3

MAN vs FOOD

Here are ways you can tidy up your man-habitat and sort out your food foraging habits so each day takes you a step closer to a smaller belly.

Home
- Quick ideas for breakfast and lunches
- What your dinner should look like
- Short cuts (for quick meals)
- Kitchen rules to play it safe
- Using leftovers
- How to beat the supermarket system
- Understand what the numbers mean on the label

Away
- Good snacks on the go
- Good lunches to buy
- Better food for the travellin' man
- What to eat when watching sport
- Mastering business dinners
- Ordering at restaurants
- Healthier meeting munchies

MAN vs FOOD—AT HOME

If you're like most men, what you do day-in and day-out is what really makes a difference to your belly-busting success. It's the cumulative effects of changes to your daily routine that really add up. The great thing about home is you can make sure that the foods in the fridge and cupboards are your friends. It's the old 'if it's healthy keep it handy' motto.

KITCHEN CLEAROUT

Take a good look at your fridge, freezer and pantry. Are these the supplies of a man who cares about his body? Are these the foods to help you fit better into your trousers? If not, cull the crap and stock up on foods to help you be a better man.

- Switch the crisps and cheesy, salty snacks for unsalted nuts (salt causes fluid retention and bloating).
- Swap the chocolate and cream biscuits for wheatmeal, oat or dried fruit-filled biscuits or fruit bread.
- Ditch the giant fatty steaks and sausages and go for smaller, leaner cuts.

EAT BREAKFAST

It doesn't need to be large, fancy, eaten at dawn or even eaten at a table—just eat it.

Breakfast food should be tasty, packed with nutritional goodies and enjoyable—start the day as you mean to continue.

Men who skip breakfast have bigger bellies.

Jump starts: quick and great tasting breakfasts

- Blend low-fat passionfruit yoghurt with low-fat milk and canned apricots for a quick smoothie. Sneak in a little wheatgerm.
- Simply combine two low-GI cereals such as bran cereal and muesli, top with sliced strawberries or bananas and

serve with low-fat fruit yoghurt or low-fat milk—or a bit of both depending how liquid you like it.
- Top your favourite muesli with plain yoghurt, maple syrup and mixed berries.
- Enjoy toasted fruit loaf spread with ricotta cheese and fruit spread.
- Zap some instant porridge in the microwave and top with sliced banana or a few sultanas.
- Toast a mixed-grain muffin and top with a slice of tomato and poached or scrambled egg.
- Whack some canned sardines or baked beans on toast.

Great starts: for when you have a bit more time
- Dip a slice or two of low-GI bread into egg whisked with low-fat milk and finely grated orange zest for French toast. Spray a pan with oil and cook the bread on each side. Serve with fresh or canned peaches or bananas and passionfruit (see page 19 for low-GI bread suggestions).
- Make or buy some small pancakes and top with ricotta cheese whisked with maple syrup and strawberries.
- Make an easy muesli by mixing oats, wheatgerm, any type of bran (wheat, rice or oats), pecans or almonds and sunflower seeds with dried apricots, sultanas, sweetened dried cranberries and chopped prunes. For extra flavour, toast the oats and nuts.
- Boil eggs and serve in egg cups with toast soldiers—an all-time fave!

EAT LUNCH
Don't get caught up in whatever you're doing and skip lunch. The hunger monster will catch up with you and strike back with a vengeance—usually after dinner when you grab for the biscuits and chocolate (the hunger monster never forgets being cheated out of a meal).

Lunches that rev up your afternoon

- Toss some chargrilled peppers and chopped red onion with burghul. Add spinach leaves, feta and basil and dress with a balsamic vinaigrette.
- Toss some shredded poached chicken with iceberg lettuce, spring onions, grated carrot, chopped coriander and vermicelli noodles. Dress with sweet chilli sauce, lime juice, fish sauce, a little sugar and peanut oil.
- Bake some sliced beetroot (it's quicker sliced than whole) and mix with spinach leaves, rocket leaves, toasted walnuts and ricotta cheese. Drizzle with oil and red wine vinegar. Serve with sourdough toast, rubbed with a garlic clove. (Tip: You can cook fresh beetroot in the microwave too.)
- Use up leftover roast sweet potato and steamed broccoli or courgettes to add to a frittata with spring onions, reduced-fat cheese and parsley. If you have any pastrami, ham or chicken, add that too.
- For a tasty soup, cook carrots or sweet potato in a little oil. Add split peas, onion, garlic, ginger and curry spices, add stock, cook and then puree. Serve with a swirl of yoghurt and mint.
- Roll up lean roast beef and tabouli with a dollop of hummus in a wrap or Lebanese bread. Or stuff into pita bread.
- Enjoy a quick, healthy sandwich of dense grainy bread filled with ham, grainy mustard, tomato and butter lettuce.

GEAR UP FOR SUCCESS

Like many endeavours, eating a good DIY lunch away from home relies on good equipment. Invest in a sturdy, good-looking lunchbox or bag that can be kept cool with an ice brick or frozen bottle of water. Have a variety of airtight, microwave-safe containers to keep foods intact and separate if required. If you can't re-heat food at work, use an insulated thermos to keep drinks, soups and stews warm. A quality stainless steel water bottle will take the rough and tumble of travel and won't degrade over time like plastic.

What is ...

Orange/lemon zest is the coloured bit (not the white pith underneath) on the outside of the skin which has loads of flavour and aroma. You can remove the zest using the fine side of a grater, or cut fine slithers using a zester (available in kitchenware shops)

Ricotta cheese is a soft Italian whey cheese much lower in fat than hard yellow cheese. You can buy it in tubs in the cheese section at supermarkets or by weight from the delicatessen counter. You can use ricotta for sweet and savoury things.

Burghul is cracked whole wheat that has been pre-cooked and only needs soaking in water before using in salads—the most famous is tabouli (a Middle Eastern parsley salad you get on a kebab). It is also known as bulgur or bulghur wheat. You can buy it near the rice, pasta and couscous in the supermarket or in delicatessens.

Pastrami is sliced beef that has been brined, smoked, seasoned and then steamed. The classic New York sandwich is pastrami on rye bread.

A **frittata** is a quiche without the pastry, or an omelette on steroids. It is made with eggs and a variety of fillings, cooked in a frypan and then the top is nicely browned under the grill.

✻ Tips for the communal kitchen at work

- Get a lunchbox or bag that fits on the shelf and put your name on it (if theft is an issue, get one that isn't see-through).
- Ask your employer to provide fruit instead of (or as well as) biscuits for staff.
- Keep some wholegrain bread, muffins or crumpets in the freezer to toast for a quick snack (hide in a coloured plastic bag if necessary).
- Store some wholegrain crackers in an airtight container to tame the hunger monster.
- If you don't have it already, request light milk be included in the office milk order.
- Keep margarine spread and toast toppings, like peanut butter, jam or yeast extract, for quick toast snacks.

DOWNSIZE YOUR DINNER

Eating too much at the end of the day is a common problem for hard-working men in demanding jobs. It's typical to work through lunch and eat like a horse at dinner and throughout the evening. This isn't helpful in the quest for a smaller belly.

To bust your belly, you need to cut down on how much you eat in the evening. The bigger the portions served up to you, the more you will eat. This is not unique to the male of the species but universally human. Make your portions smaller. This is tough at first but becomes easier over time.

Great dinners

- Bake some salmon fillets smeared with sweet chilli sauce and ginger and serve on a bed of soba noodles mixed with spring onions, toasted sesame seeds, mint and shredded carrot.
- Marinate some lean loin chops in curry powder, ginger, garlic, lemon juice and a little oil. Grill or barbecue them and serve with a rice pilaf made with basmati rice, onion, curry powder, red peppers and peas.
- Marinate chicken cubes in tandoori paste and yoghurt. Skewer and barbecue. Serve with a salad of tomato, cucumber, spring onions, chickpeas, mint, parsley and lemon juice.
- Pan-fry onions, peppers, mushrooms and Mexican spices (eg, paprika, oregano, cumin and chilli). Throw in a can of tomatoes and canned (drained) lentils. Spoon into tortillas, roll them up and serve with an easy salsa of kidney beans, corn, spring onions, fresh coriander and lime juice.
- For a quick pasta sauce, fry an onion, chopped lean bacon and thyme in a little olive oil. Throw in mushrooms and finish with spinach, parsley, ricotta and balsamic vinegar.

- Bake a pork fillet marinated in char sieu sauce. Slice over stir-fried onions, ginger, snow peas and wombok (Chinese cabbage) with low-GI rice.
- Enjoy a healthy beef stroganoff by adding lots of onions and mushrooms, using less lean beef strips and extending reduced-fat sour cream with a flavoursome sauce of chicken stock, Dijon mustard, paprika and tomato paste.

What is...

Soba noodles are Japanese noodles made from a combination of buckwheat flour and regular wheat flour, giving them a light brown-grey colour.

Pilaf is a mixed dish of rice, vegetables and seasoning, with or without meat.

Basmati is a fragrant variety of rice traditionally used in Indian cooking. It has a moderate GI—why it's a belly-busting ally.

Tandoori paste is a blend of traditional Indian spices combined with oil.

Salsa is a Spanish word for sauce and means anything you can serve with plain food to make it tasty (and it doesn't even need to be liquid). There are plenty available in the supermarket, such as tomato-based Mexican style with chilli.

Char sieu is Chinese barbecue sauce usually used with pork.

Balsamic vinegar is a traditional Italian vinegar made from sweet white wine that has been matured in wooden barrels to give it a dark colour and rich flavour.

GET THE CUPS OUT

You've gotta measure it to really control the portions. You can buy sets of measuring cups (1 cup, 1/3 cup, 1/2 cup, 1/4 cup) in supermarkets and kitchen tool shops. Get a set of spoons (1 tablespoon, 1 teaspoon, 1/2 teaspoon) while you're there.

Show and tell

Here's what typical main meals should actually look like. Taking your cup in hand, Medium to Large men stick to one cup of carbs (pasta, noodles); Extra Large men can have two cups (or stick to one and bust your belly faster).

- 1–2 cups of al dente pasta with 1–2 cups of vegetable-rich bolognaise sauce and a salad with dressing (see page 156).
- ½–1 cup of cooked rice with about ½–1 cup of stir-fried meat or chicken strips and at least 1½ cups of vegetables (the more the better).
- 1–2 cups of noodles, 1 or 2 eggs and a combination of Asian stir-fried vegetables.
- 1 roast chicken quarter (without skin) served with 1–2 medium-sized baked potatoes (or similar-sized sweet potato) plus at least 1 cup of other vegetables such as peas, beans, broccoli and cauliflower.
- 4 regular-sized taco shells filled with chilli beans, lettuce, tomato slices, grated reduced fat cheese and ¼ avocado.
- 1–2 multigrain muffins or bread rolls spread with grainy or Dijon mustard and topped with 1–2 grilled hamburger patties and tomato and cucumber slices, lettuce, onion rings, beetroot and grated carrot.

BEWARE OF THE SQUARE-EYED JUNK MONSTER
Eating while watching TV is a bad idea—you will eat mindlessly (probably fattening food), plus your metabolic rate (fuel-burning ability) slows right down to a level not much higher than sleeping.

If you must have an 'extra' food treat, have it during the day and eat a little less of something else. For example, if you have a hankering for a bag of crisps, make it a small bag and reduce the size of your lunch. Enjoy them more because you have them less often (and eat them slowly).

SHORT CUTS—FROZEN, CANNED, PACKETS

You may be lucky enough to have someone else cook for you, but when that's not possible there are shortcuts to enjoying belly-busting meals.

Frozen meals from the supermarket are a great standby and ready in a few minutes. Buy ones that are labelled 'low fat', 'healthier' or 'lean'. Bonus points for microwaving some extra frozen veggies to go with it or making a side salad.

For a bigger appetite, have a wholemeal or mixed grain roll with the meal as well. These work well for office lunches too, and are competitively priced compared to takeaway meals.

Home-delivered meals that are good for belly busting are available. You can have all your meals, or just dinners, delivered. They've done the hard work for you by crunching the kilojoules and ensuring the food is good to eat and good for you.

This method is a no-brainer for men who don't cook, but remember it's good to learn how to feed yourself properly in the long run. You can't rely on others your whole life.

Meal-makers are products from the supermarket that transform meat and vegetables into a meal. Examples include recipe mixes, pasta sauces, stir-fry sauces, pasta and sauce, instant sauces and the like. Sure, there is compromise to be made on salt content (you can look for reduced-salt versions), but on balance these make meals that are streets ahead of 'quick and dirty' home delivery or drive-thru. And you get to say 'I made it myself'.

To bust your belly, avoid eating or drinking beer or soft drinks, etc. in front of the TV—especially as treats. Have a cup of tea, coffee, light hot chocolate or diet soft drink/cordial instead.

If you can't make it, fake it!

Here are a few quick and easy meal ideas using convenience products.

Fasta pasta Pasta + lean mince + vegetables (onion, garlic, peppers, aubergine, mushroom) + bottled pasta sauce + fresh basil leaves + sprinkle of parmesan.

Using your noodle Quick low-fat noodles + can of flavoured tuna + frozen peas and corn + chopped parsley.

Curry in a hurry Chicken breast + curry paste + veggies (onion, garlic, carrot, capsicum, chickpeas, frozen peas, zucchini) + coconut-flavoured evaporated milk + fresh coriander leaves.

Super speedy stir-fry Lean beef strips + vegetables (onion, garlic, ginger, carrot, celery, peppers, courgettes—or frozen stir-fry vegetable mix) + stir-fry sauce + 90-second rice.

Bonza burritos Soft flour tortillas + chilli beef and beans in a can + Mexican salsa in a jar + light natural yoghurt + mixed salad in a bag.

WAIST NOT, WASTE NOT—REVIVING LEFTOVERS

The amount of food we waste is a national shame and environmental disaster. Our parents and grandparents were far more frugal with food and we need to bring back this habit, not only to save money and save the planet but because it helps bust your belly too. If you know how to revive leftovers, you can whip up a meal in a flash and are less likely to dial a pizza. You'll also save money.

Single serves is a good way of saving leftovers—that means spooning enough for one person into each container. This makes microwave re-heating simple and controls the amount you (and others) eat. Stackable microwave-safe containers reheat more quickly and fit better in the fridge or freezer.

What to do with leftover ...

Rice: Make fried rice with egg and vegetables; mix with flavoured tuna and chopped tomato and parsley; use as a base for curry or stir-fry.

Pasta: Make a pasta salad with three-bean mix, vegetables and dressing; a pasta bake using a low-fat bottled sauce using the recipe on the jar; toss through some canned salmon, lemon juice, green peas and fresh dill.

Barbecue chicken: Chicken and corn soup; chicken, avocado, mayonnaise and salad wrap; green chicken curry (with coconut-flavoured evaporated milk).

Roast meat: Sandwiches and wraps; curry and rice; minestrone soup.

Potatoes: Potato salad with mayonnaise and chopped fresh herbs; with onion in a potato omelette or frittata; in vegetable soup.

Thai curry: Serve with freshly cooked noodles and extra vegetables; use as a sauce for cooked meat, chicken or fish.

Chinese: Serve with freshly cooked rice and extra vegetables; filling for toasted sandwich or wrap; add to soup.

Steak: Steak sandwich or burger; chop up for casserole or curry; top with warmed salsa, a slice of light cheese and grill.

We eat with our eyes as well as our mouths. Even if you're zapping a frozen meal in the microwave, serve it up at the table and sit down and enjoy it properly. Eat slowly and you're bound to feel more satisfied than inhaling it while standing over the bench.

Not wasting food is all part of your new belly-busting mindset of treating food and your body with respect. Buy and eat the quality food that your body needs.

Man vs Food

KITCHEN RULES
Play it safe
Make sure food is handled correctly to avoid food poisoning. Food is not only nourishing for you but also to bacteria. You need to make life hard for bugs with good kitchen hygiene and temperature control.

Clean up your act
Always wash your hands with soap and running water before you start cooking, and between handling raw and cooked foods—raw foods (especially chicken) are covered in bacteria. Wipe down your benches with hot soapy water (antibacterial products are not necessary). Keep all your utensils clean. Avoid smelly bacteria-laden dish cloths by regularly washing or disinfecting—you can throw them in the washing machine.

Prevent cross-contamination
The bacteria from raw foods can jump across to ready-to-eat foods and into your mouth if you're not careful. Have separate equipment (knives and chopping boards) for raw foods, or ensure you wash them with hot soapy water before using for ready-to-eat food, such as salad or bread. Never pour marinades from raw meat onto cooked meat.

Control the temperature
- Keep food out of the balmy bacteria danger zone: between 5°C (40°F) and 60°C (140°F).
- Ensure your fridge is at 4°C (39.2°F)—invest in a fridge thermometer.
- Don't leave chilled foods out of the fridge too long. Put cold stuff used in cooking back in the fridge before sitting down to a meal.
- Ensure your raw meat, chicken and fish is well contained to prevent juices dripping onto other foods—a dish covered with plastic wrap or a takeaway container works well.

SIZE CONTROL

If you've made too much, serve out the extra into a container straightaway (like dishing out for an extra person) to stop you eating it.

- When re-heating foods, ensure they are steaming hot all the way through (stir during heating).
- Put leftovers into the fridge as soon as the steam stops (no need to wait until they are cool) and eat them within two to three days. If you can't eat them this quickly, freeze them.
- Don't keep food that has been standing around at room temperature for more than two hours (for example, foods at a barbecue). Put the leftovers in the fridge as soon as you've finished and you've got another meal half-made for the next day.

CRUISING THE AISLES

Navigating the supermarket needs sound strategy and planning. Remember, they're not designed to be your belly-busting ally. They are actually designed to prey on the hapless and harried shopper with all kinds of clever techniques. Their aim is to get you to buy more than you need and, in some sections such as the breakfast aisle, more highly processed sugar-laden foods than are good for you.

✳ Shopping tips

- Keep a shopping list on or near your fridge and add to it through the week—take it with you to avoid impulse buys.
- Buy mostly from around the edges of the supermarket— this is where most of the foods you need to eat (meat, chicken, fish, milk, yoghurt, cheese, fruit and vegetables) are located. The centre aisles tend to be a carnival of party food and other fattening and unhealthy fare.
- When you head for the centre (looking for canned vegetables or fish or pasta or rice), do not depart from your list.
- Before you get in the checkout queue, check out your trolley contents and imagine your plate. In general, do you

BEAT THE SYSTEM

Like finding your way around a new town, in a supermarket you need to know exactly where you want to go (ie, have a clear destination) and a have good map. Your destination is a smaller belly; your map is your shopping list.

SUPERMARKET STRATEGIES

- They put products they want you to buy at eye level and at the ends of the aisles—these are not necessarily the foods you need to eat or are good for you—look high and low for 'reduced-salt', 'high-fibre' and 'low-fat' products.
- They tempt you with sweet treats at the checkout.
- They convince you to buy food you don't want with price discounts.
- They make you walk past heaps of stuff you don't need on the way to the stuff you do.

have mostly vegetables, fruits, grain foods and legumes; moderate amounts of lean meat and dairy foods, and small amounts of extra or treat foods? (It's fun to check out other people's trolleys too!)

NOTE: Meal-maker products that help to put together healthy balanced meals fall in the 'eat moderately' category too.

SUPPLY MANAGEMENT

Achieving your belly-busting goal requires stocking your kitchen with the right food. If it's there, you'll eat it. Conversely, if it's not there, you can't eat it (or at least you have to go out of your way to eat it—and have time to think about whether you really want to).

In psychological lingo, only buying the food you want to eat is called pre-commitment and is an effective way to achieve a smaller belly.

KNOWING YOUR NUMBERS
Percent guideline daily amount (%GDA) for adults is 2000 calories, although the average man needs 2500 calories. Despite this, %GDAs offer a reasonable target for belly-busting men.

There are %GDAs for different nutrients:

- calories
- sugars
- fat
- saturated fat (saturates)
- sodium (salt)

How to use the %GDA numbers

- Look for lower %GDA numbers in everything except fibre and protein.
- For calories a meal should be about 25%GDA (if you eat three meals and two snacks in a day). A large-sized burger from a fast-food chain is over 20%GDA of an average man—and that's before you even think about fries or a drink. A large meal deal of burger, fries and cola is around a whopping 50%GDA—way too much unless you can eat very little at other meals.
- Any %GDA is too much for a drink (unless it's low-fat milk and you're having it as a hot or cold liquid snack). Zero sugar drinks and tea and coffee without sugar have virtually zero %GDA.
- Any snack with more than 10%GDA is too much—100g (3½oz) dark chocolate is 20%GDA whereas an oat muesli bar with nuts is under 10%.

NUMBER CRUNCH

Quite a few food manufacturers have elected to use a nutrition labelling system called Guideline Daily Amount, or %GDA. You'll see these as 'thumbnails' on food packages; either a single calorie thumbnail (like on a can of soft drink) or multiple thumbnails (as on breakfast cereal boxes). The %GDA is the percentage of the daily recommended total for adults in a serving of the food.

MAN vs FOOD—AWAY

So many men say they eat pretty well when they're in domestic captivity. It's braving the fattening world outside that trips them up. Here are strategies to cope with high-risk situations and equip yourself with the skills to bust your belly no matter where you are.

SNACKS ON THE GO

The first question to ask is, are you really hungry? If the answer is no, don't eat anything and have some water or a diet drink instead.

Eating when you're not even hungry will add to the size of your belly rather than bust it. It's a seriously unhelpful habit. Before you eat anything, you need to practise asking yourself, 'Am I hungry, and how hungry am I?' and eat (or not) accordingly. Say no to being led by the nose by snack-food companies who want you to eat more than you need and to eat food you'd be better off without.

If you are hungry, focus on the key foods your body needs. Snacks are just top-ups of healthy foods eaten in smaller amounts. Think of them as mini-meals, not an excuse to eat party food in the middle of the afternoon.

Snack foods hungry blokes need to eat

Remember to keep it small or you'll eat more than you need to bust your belly.

- **Fruit: fresh, dried, canned**—for example, bananas, dried apricots, canned fruit salad (not juice, drink water instead).
- **Light milk and yoghurt**—for example, glass of milk, tub of yoghurt, skim milkshake/smoothie, skim cafe latte/hot chocolate.
- **Wholegrain bread**—for example, bread or toast with spread, roll or sandwich or wrap, crispbread and topping, oat- or wholegrain-based muesli bar.
- **Nuts etc**—unsalted, raw or roasted (handful or two only), nut bar, roasted chickpeas, plain popcorn.

Wet vs dry

When it comes to belly busting, remember: wet foods beat dry foods. Allow me to explain ...

Foods with high water content have fewer calories by weight—they fill you up without a high calorie cost. Dry foods on the other hand are densely packed with calories and disappointingly unfulfilling. Soup is great, biscuits are not.

A simple example to illustrate the point is the potato. A boiled potato is super-filling and low in kilojoules whereas a bag of potato crisps cops quite a kilojoule wallop and is like eating air (which is why you feel you can't get enough):

1 large boiled potato—753kJ (180 calories)—satisfaction high

100g (3½oz) bag potato chips—2130kJ (509 calories)—satisfaction low

It is similar with rice versus rice crackers. Don't be conned by 'baked not fried' and 'low fat' claims on things like crackers, savoury biscuits and the like. These are terribly more-ish, low in nutrition and frighteningly fattening whether baked or fried—and think of the toppings and dips that come along with them for the ride.

Drink think. Don't even think about purchasing a regular soft drink. A 375ml (12fl oz) can of cola contains ten teaspoons of sugar. If you must, choose a zero sugar option. Although fruit juices are obviously healthier, they contain the same amount of sugar and kilojoules so give them a miss to bust your belly.

You might have heard that eating every few hours is a good thing, and the word 'metabolism' was probably mentioned. Forget it. Your body does not burn fat any differently whether you eat three times a day or six—it's how much you eat in total that counts. If it helps you to eat smaller meals with snacks in between, do it (and choose well). If you don't need to snack, don't—it's helpful in your quest to eat less.

MEN'S WISDOM

Geoff, aged 60, retired
My waist size is a worry because of the health implications, the way it limits my physical abilities and the negative effects on my wardrobe. What has helped me is to take active holidays with friends who like camping and bushwalking. You've got to maintain friendships with friends who are also interested in exercising and being active.

LUNCH ON THE GO

So you're in your local food court or shopping strip—what do you buy? Luckily, our united nations of cuisine provides heaps of choice.

Good choices include:

Italian: Pasta with primavera (vegetable and tomato sauce), marinara (but choose a tomato-based seafood sauce not a creamy one) or puttanesca sauce (garlic, olives, capers and chilli). Skip the garlic bread and lasagne.

Japanese: Sushi, sashimi, stir-fry and rice or noodle. Skip the tempura.

Mexican: Rice or burritos with chilli beef and beans. Skip the cheese and sour cream.

Thai: Stir-fry and steamed rice, beef salad. Skip the fried entrees and creamy curries.

Chinese: Stir-fry and steamed rice. Skip the sweet and sour or anything with 'honey'.

Salad bar: Greens with beans plus chicken, salmon or tuna. Dressing is fine.

Sandwich bar: Wholemeal roll, sandwich or wrap with chicken, egg, salmon, tuna or roast beef and heaps of salad. Skip the cheesy focaccia.

Filled roll chain: Low-fat options (no extra cheese). Skip the extra long size and cookies for dessert.

General takeaway shop: Plain burger with salad. Skip the bacon and cheese.

Lebanese: Kebab or felafel wrap.

Fish and chip shop: Grilled fish, salad and wedges. Skip the greasy battered fish and skinny fries.

Fried chicken: Grilled chicken burger with corn cob and coleslaw.

Burger chain: Small burger, fish burger, vege-burger or wrap. Skip the fries (or have small size only), nuggets, shakes and desserts.

> Say no to large 'value' meals –where's the value in adding extra around your waist?

Read carefully

Some fast-food joints are putting the kilojoule and calorie values next to items on their menu because of government regulations. Others put nutrition information on their packaging, in brochures inside the store or on their website. Once you realise how big the numbers are, you'll want to choose more carefully. Remember, the average adult daily kilojoule/calorie requirements are 8700/2078.

PLANES, TRAINS AND AUTOMOBILES

Airports, train stations and petrol stations seem to serve food from a previous era—before the advent of motorised transport. Their tempting selection of chocolate bars, crisps, doughnuts and pies contain enough food energy for you to walk to your next destination carrying a 30kg (65lb) pack. If you're taking the sedentary transport option, don't eat them. On the up side, they are great places to be trapped in a disaster—you'll survive for months.

TRAVELLIN' LIGHT

Many men travel for work and this makes it harder to maintain a healthy food routine. If you're a travellin' man, don't let your belly be a sign you've given up on trying to eat sensibly. There are almost always healthier options available—you just need to look for them. Think before you order the usual on auto-pilot— you need a new 'usual'.

Sit down, relax and take the time to enjoy your meal—you want quick food, not quick eating.

On the road

Road food can be a nutritional nightmare but try to see past the deep-fried nasties and look for the healthier options. Avoid ordering large portions too. Opt for sandwiches, basic burgers (skip the bacon, cheese and other extras), roast meat and vegetables, noodles and stir-fries with steamed rice.

In the air

Luckily the size of in-flight meals is small. On short flights, resist the urge to purchase high-kilojoule chips, biscuits, bars and cakes (are you hungry or bored?). Try taking some fruit and water and reading a book or magazine instead. If you have to buy from the cart get a sandwich, wrap, soup, breakfast drink or muesli bar.

A SPORTING CHANCE—FOOTY SNACKS AND SPORT HAMPERS

In general, men like sport, and sporting venues tend to offer very unsporting food choices (although things are gradually changing). Depending on your situation, you'll either be dealing with corporate box excess, munching it with the masses on overpriced pies and crisps, or deciding between slim pickings at the local park kiosk. And it is highly likely there'll be pressure to drink a lot of alcohol.

Even if you play sport yourself (or go and watch your kids), the tradition of going to the pub afterwards cancels out any belly-busting benefit from the huffing and puffing. For you to get ahead in the belly-busting game, something has to change.

Unfortunately sport has become associated with alcohol and fattening food.

✷ Sports food tips
DIY

- Take a cool box with your own food and drink (this saves money as well). Pack sandwiches, wraps, chicken legs and hardboiled eggs—food that's easy to eat with your hands—plus fruit, nuts and water or diet cordial.
- Take light beer, and only how many you want to drink—when you're out, you're out. This will also help manage blood alcohol limits for driving.
- For big-bellied men there is no safety in numbers; you'll just all end up in the same hospital with heart attack, diabetes, cancer, back problems and knee reconstructions.

CHOICES

Poor	Better
Meat pie	Hot dog
Potato crisps	Hot chips
Pizza	Plain burger
Fish 'n' chips	Noodles

Man vs Food

FRIENDS OR SABOTEURS?

If drinking light beer and eating healthier food will attract scrutiny from your friends, you have to ask: what kind of friends want you to keep your big belly? It's often the kind who wants you to stay big so they can feel better about their own belly. Don't become the victim of sabotage.

MEN'S WISDOM

Rick, aged 35, teacher
I don't like my belly at all and I haven't been very successful at losing it. My suspicion is this is due to a lack of sleep, insufficient water, ineffective exercise (I can't do high-impact exercise because of injuries) and Saturday night binges after sport that undo all my good work.

IN THE KITCHEN AT PARTIES ...

Whether it's the silly season or whenever, if you attend lots of catered functions or meetings there's a risk of overdoing it on food and booze. Remember, just because it's offered to you on a platter doesn't mean you have to take it.

If you know you're prone to pig out at parties, don't turn up hungry and don't stand near the food table.

Avoid nibbles in pastry or deep-fried (be suspicious of anything golden), and keep track of how many small items you eat—they can add up to more than your usual meal. If possible fill your plate once only (or twice if the plate's tiny). Keep track of how much alcohol you drink and stop at one or two glasses—switch to diet soft drink or sparking water.

Clubhouse rules

Men getting together to share common interests or goals is a wonderful thing—whether it's to play darts, build the community or build furniture. However, the shared table over which you solve the problems of the world creates a whole world of other problems because of the food you choose.

- Who says you always need to order pizza—why not order sushi?
- When asked to bring snacks, who says you have to bring crisps and soft drink?
- For goodness sake, some of the most famous men in the media right now are chefs! Surely it's time to raise the bar. The next time you spend quality time communing with friends, try to eat better food.

MASTERING THE BUSINESS LUNCH OR DINNER

Eating in restaurants frequently as part of your work can be a slippery slope to a bigger wardrobe, especially if getting tipsy is part of your schmoozing strategy. It's amazing how many men have told me how competitive eating and drinking can be. It's almost medieval how overeating and drinking can symbolise power and influence among men. It's also easy to see why many successful men have big bellies. This power game over the restaurant table is akin to digging your own grave with a knife and fork. Step up to the plate and change the rules—make it OK to eat and drink lightly and you'll give other men permission to do the same.

✶ Restaurant tips

- Don't turn up starving—try having a glass of light milk or banana beforehand (you cannot expect to eat lightly with the hunger beast on your back).
- Have a tall glass of water before you order, and drink more water with your meal.
- Order one course only, or two entrees.
- Order using the half-quarter-quarter plate principle; half your plate vegetables or salad, one quarter meat, chicken or fish and one quarter carbohydrates (pasta, bread, rice or noodles)—see page 166.
- Order extra vegetables or salad if need be (many restaurants do not automatically serve vegetables with 'meals', although calling a vegetable-free dish a meal is a stretch).
- Avoid anything deep-fried, wrapped in pastry or with a cream and/or butter sauce.
- Choose grilled, steamed, stir-fried or baked dishes.
- Skip the bread on the side or, if you must, have plain bread rather than oily garlic/herb.
- Skip alcohol, or limit yourself to one or two glasses.

- Skip dessert and move straight to coffee, or share a dessert (sometimes a taste is all you need to satisfy your sweet tooth).

BETTER BUSINESS MEETINGS

Whether it's a training workshop, board meeting or strategy conference, ask the meeting organiser to request healthier catering. It's madness to serve up huge amounts of kilojoule-laden food and drinks when you've been couped up inside on your backside all day. Eating lighter food will also boost productivity rather than send everyone to sleep.

A heavy meal diverts blood to the gut for digestion rather than to the brain for thinking. Choose lighter food to boost brain power.

Better meeting munchies
- Antipasto (olives, artichoke hearts, marinated vegetables)
- Vegetable sticks, pita bread and dips
- Sushi
- Meat or chicken skewers
- Chargrilled vegetable skewers
- Meatballs and salsa
- Frittata
- Barbecued chicken without skin
- Prawns and oysters
- Sandwiches and wraps
- Steamed dim sum
- Rice paper rolls
- Noodle boxes
- Fruit platter.

Men's wisdom

Martin, aged 57, CEO marketing company

Considering I spend so much time at work, I thought it was time to get our office in order. I did it because I'm interested in health and wellbeing and because we look after a lot of heath-related clients. It just looked bad when we served up cakes and biscuits to health, fitness and health food clients.

We've cleaned up our act and now serve fruit, sandwiches and wraps, and chilled water. We don't buy soft drinks and have a 'no-alcohol' policy for business lunches. We got rid of the bowls of sweets from the boardroom table and only order light milk for tea and coffee. We also get a box of fresh fruit delivered every week—the staff really appreciate that. There was grumbling at first but now everyone is used to the idea they can see the benefits. Several staff say they've lost a bit of weight. It was just the right thing to do.

PART 4

CONQUER THE KITCHEN & SHRINK YOUR BELLY

In this section are all the recipes I have created, tested and eaten so you can cook and eat the foods your body needs in portions to help bust your belly. Conquering the kitchen is an important step in taking control of the food you eat and a great opportunity to impress with your cooking skills (without the years of training).

The recipe content has been designed to share basic preparation, cooking and serving skills to make cooking easy, fun and rewarding in every way. The flavours of the dishes are gutsy, using lots of aromatic spices, fresh fragrant herbs, a variety of meat, fish, eggs, fresh, frozen and canned vegetables, fresh and dried fruits and a selection of grains and breads. I have adapted popular ethnic dishes into everyday eating recipes that took my tastebuds while creating them to places I'd only every dreamed of going—hopefully they'll do the same for you.

The recipes tips and options give you the scope to personalise the recipes to your taste. Please experiment and try something new—you may be pleasantly surprised. Always taste as you go while cooking and don't be afraid to add a little bit more of this or that as long as it is on the ingredient list—at least the first time you try the recipe.

No salt has been included in the recipes and the delicious real food flavours will linger in your mouth rather than an overpowering saltiness as if you've just swallowed a mouthful of seawater.

You've taken the time to cook up a great meal so take the time to savour every morsel.

The shared table always adds to the enjoyment of a meal. However, if you are eating alone don't just gobble it down in a hurry. Set a place at the table, eat slowly and experience the textures and flavour of every bite. Taking time to eat may be a new experience for you but it's a new habit that's well worth taking on. The enjoyment of the food and the satisfaction of having cooked a belly-busting meal is something to be proud of.

Go on, have a go and try out the recipes: there is something for everyone. There are recipes for one, two or four people. There are simple ideas just assembling ingredients, easy barbecues, popular fast-food meals, recipes for all day eating and some fancy fare that will impress. Imagine how good you'll feel when you've cooked up something to share and you can say 'I made it myself' when strutting your new more streamlined physique.

Have fun!

GETTING INTO GEAR: THE RIGHT TOOLS FOR THE JOB

Oven, cooktops and griller Often these are already chosen for us, but if you do have a choice when building or doing a kitchen renovation, thoroughly research the options, talk to the sales experts and if possible attend some cooking demonstrations. They are big-ticket items and you need to get it right the first time. You deserve the best your budget can manage and for your enjoyment when cooking.

Microwave oven Do you want it to be simple or slick, single function or multi-functional, cheap as chips or top dollar? Again, do some homework: it really is a minefield when it comes to microwave ovens and will depend on what will suit your needs best. Mostly, you just want to zap food until it's hot, so a basic model will be ideal. If you need it to grill and bake too, choose a combo oven, put on your L plate and go and have some lessons—many microwave oven manufacturers hold classes or in-store demonstrations so take yourself off to one or two and you'll soon be more than qualified.

Barbecue Basically there are two types: uncovered or covered. An uncovered barbecue is more traditional but the covered barbecue is more versatile because you can use it as an oven.

There are a number of things to consider when buying a barbecue. Will you be cooking for small or large numbers? Is it for a huge outdoor area or a small balcony? Would you want to use it as an oven? Do you only require something basic or do you need a more elaborate barbecue? Go to the barbecue specialists, attend demonstrations and tastings and ask lots of questions.

Food processor, blender or mixer A kitchen can't be without one. It can be large or small—you may need one of each or it can be a multi-functional appliance, the choice will depend on your cooking requirements. The best stick blenders are extremely versatile so are worth considering before you invest in an expensive machine you may not use much. Combined with a really good knife (see below), you may not need anything else.

Kitchen must-haves

Resist the temptation to fill up your cupboards and cover the benches with unnecessary kitchen gadgets—good practical tools do numerous jobs and a piece of equipment that only performs one task can easily become redundant.

Cutting knives A set in a knife block can look fantastic on the bench but they need to do more than just look good. Knives need to be kept sharp, feel balanced in your hand and be appropriate for what you need to do. If you go for a set in a knife block, choose a reputable brand. Take every opportunity to test family and friends' knives before you purchase your own—you'll get a feel for the knives that you find comfortable and as the same time do a good job.

If your choice is not to buy a knife set, essential needs are:

- an all-purpose chef/cook's knife; blades vary from 15–25cm (6–10in)
- two paring knives, one with a serrated edge, blade length about 10cm (4in)
- a bread knife with a serrated edge blade 15–22cm (6–9in)
- a knife sharpening steel or a stone.

Pans Be guided by the size of your cooktops as to the size of the saucepans and frying pans you'll need. Invest in heavy-based pans and the best quality you can afford. Pans can last for decades so good quality is good economy. Pans are always a great buy when the major stores have the kitchenware sales. Buying pans individually is recommended—you can always add extra if needed.

Good purchases would be:

- non-stick saucepan and frying pan, with a base of 165–18cm (6–7in). If they're the same size, you can use the saucepan lid on the frying pan
- non-stick saucepan and frying pan, each with a base of 20–28cm (8–11in). Again, you can use the saucepan lid on both
- heavy ovenproof casserole with a lid to use on the cooktop and in the oven—one with a base of 22cm (9in) is very versatile
- non-stick wok with a lid
- roasting pan with a rack, the size depending on the size of your oven
- heavy griller pan to sit on the cooktop—this could be round or rectangular. It may sit on one cooktop or across two—be guided by your stove top as to the shape and size that would be the most practical for your needs. A combination grill and flat plate can be handy for achieving the fantastic flavour and cool-looking stripes chargrilling gives to food, and you can cook eggs, fritters and pancakes on the flat plate. It's like bringing the barbecue indoors.

Chopping boards Consider buying a set of different coloured cutting boards to help eliminate cross-contamination of food. You could use separate boards for red meat, poultry and seafood, remembering never to use the same one for cooked meat that was used for cutting up raw meat. Use another board for dairy foods and one for fruit and vegetables. But you really only need one or two, washed after using with different ingredients—use one for meats, fish etc plus onions and garlic and other vegetables; the other for anything you absolutely don't want tainted with onion, garlic, fish smells, etc. A wooden board is perfect for slicing bread—a good-looking one always looks great at the table.

OTHER EQUIPMENT ESSENTIALS

- Balloon whisk
- Can opener
- Colander
- Fish slice
- Garlic crusher, if you are into gadgets—smashing garlic on a board with the blade of a knife is better.
- Kitchen scissors
- Oven mitts
- Potato masher
- Silicon spatulas for non-stick cookware
- Slotted spoon
- Stainless steel mixing bowls
- Strainer/sieve, large and small
- Tongs
- Wooden spoons

Grater A good stainless steel box grater with a handle is ideal for slicing, zesting, coarse and fine grating and shredding. A small handheld grater is good for parmesan cheese; ones called microplanes are available for fine and coarse grating and are exceptionally good.

Peeler A good strong vegetable peeler is a great asset and takes the frustration out of attacking difficult hard-skinned vegetables, as well as more pliable potatoes and the like.

Measuring cups and spoons A set of standard measuring cups and spoons and a liquid measuring cup are a must—don't take chances with quantities but measure for accuracy.

PANTRY ESSENTIALS

Try not to overstock the pantry—remember that foods have best-before dates. It is much more economical to use up what's in the pantry before buying up big on bargains and then ultimately throwing away all the out-of-date products. See the Cupboard hunt section (pages 137–42) for great ideas for using up pantry stock.

Cereal and oats Try wheat or oat breakfast biscuits, wholegrain bran or oat cereal, traditional oats or the Raisin, cranberry and walnut grain-ola mix that you've made yourself.

Good oils Choose sunflower, canola or rice bran oil for everyday cooking and extra virgin olive oil for salad dressings and tossing lightly through cooked vegetables as a 'good for you' finishing flavour booster. It is a good idea to keep an eye on the best-before date and discard oil if it has passed its use-by date.

Balsamic vinegar Buy good-quality aged balsamic vinegar—a little goes a long way and it really livens up the flavour of food and dressings.

Worcestershire sauce It's been around forever and still there's nothing to compare with it—a dash in stews, casseroles and sauces rounds off and sharpens flavours.

Beans Stock canned salt-reduced baked beans, canned and dried kidney and cannellini beans.

Lentils and chickpeas Buy both canned and dried.

Tomatoes Have canned whole peeled, diced or chopped with no added salt.

DATE MARKING OF FOODS
A use-by date appears on perishable foods that may not be safe to eat after this date. A best-before date is a recommendation for quality. You can still eat foods after their best-before date but their quality may have declined. For example, they may not be as crunchy, or some flavour may be lost.

Herbs and spices Not too many—just keep your favourites and blends. Must-haves for these recipes are smoked paprika, cinnamon and sumac, garam masala, bought or homemade baharat and dukkah (see recipes, pages 152–53).

Pasta and rice Choose wholemeal pasta and low-GI rice as healthy all-rounders and for speedy rice use brown 90-second microwave rice.

Noodles Dry rice vermicelli noodles are useful.

Salmon, tuna and sardines Buy slices or whole, canned in spring water.

Stock Use powdered or liquid, salt-reduced.

FRIDGE ESSENTIALS

If there are only good things in the fridge then your choices will be healthy ones.

Dairy Buy low- or reduced-fat milk and yoghurt.

Cheese Keep a small quantity of good parmesan and reduced-fat cheddar.

Spread Choose salt-reduced sunflower or canola margarine spread.

Mayonnaise Choose a good-quality one that ideally is low in sodium.

Nuts Keep a supply of different types of nuts in the fridge—they'll keep better. Dry-roast the nuts over a very low heat in a non-stick pan until they smell really toasty and nutty, then cool before eating—they'll taste sensational.

Fruit and vegetables Keep them in the crisper drawer of the fridge. Wrapping them in plastic bags will prevent them drying out and they'll last longer; wrap delicate vegetables in paper towels to prevent them going slimy. Stone fruits are best taken out of the fridge and brought to back room temperature for optimum flavour enjoyment. Tomatoes are best stored at room temperature—ie, out of the fridge.

Eggs They'll keep fresh longer when stored in their carton in the fridge.

FREEZER ESSENTIALS

Everyone has a freezer and it's not only for ice and ice cream. It can be such a good friend when you're really hungry and there is a complete frozen meal that you can just whip out, thaw and heat in the microwave, or some vegetables to complete a meal and make it nutritionally balanced.

Leftovers Make the most when cooking up meals and do an extra portion. Place it in a freezer-proof container, wait until the steam stops and seal, label and date and freeze.

Vegetables Peas, mixed vegetables and single-serve microwavable packs are in convenient packs. It's a good idea to flatten them out and stack them flat so you don't have to wrestle with clumps of frozen vegetables. If you buy in bulk separating and storing in single-sized portions is a great idea and any leftover roast vegetables are perfect for freezing.

Fruit Commercial frozen products are excellent and great to thaw and add to breakfast cereal and yoghurt or to use as a base for a crumble. Frozen berries and overripe frozen bananas make super-thick smoothies made with skim or low-fat milk. If a banana is too ripe to eat fresh, you can put the whole thing in the freezer—the skin will turn black but the inside will still be good.

Ice cream and frozen yoghurt Make sure that it is low or reduced fat.

Ice A glass (or jug) full of fresh ice cubes, filled with water, freshly squeezed lemon or lime juice and a few slices of lemon or lime on a hot day is an amazing thirst quencher and hunger deterrent.

HELPFUL GUIDE TO FREEZING TIMES

Food	Freezing times (maximum recommendations)
Beef—raw	
steaks and roasts	6 months
mince	3 months
Lamb—raw	
cutlets and roasts	6 months
mince	3 months
Chicken—raw	
whole	12 months
pieces	6 months
mince	3 months
Pork—raw	
chops and roasts	3–6 months
mince	2 months
bacon	1 month
Seafood—raw	
fish fillets (white)	6 months
oily fillets (salmon or trout)	2 months
shellfish	2 months
Fruits and vegetables—frozen	Check 'best-before' date on packet
Casseroles—cooked	
beef and lamb	3 months
pork	1 month
vegetarian	6 months
Soups—cooked	4 months

GOOD TO KNOW

Things to help make using the recipes in this book and cooking a little easier.

What's 'roughly chopped'? Small and large irregular shapes—there's no need to be too fussy.

What's 'finely chopped'? More time and precision is needed for chopping as it may be very important for the cooking time and the texture of the finished dish.

'Preheat the oven'? The oven does need to be at a particular temperature when something goes in to be cooked but it doesn't need hours of preheating. You need to get in tune with your oven. Most ovens have a light that goes off when the set temperature has been reached; take note as to whether it needs 5 or 10 minutes to heat up or longer and use this as a guide for when to turn on your oven.

Conventional oven temperature or fan-forced? Whatever works best for you; if you prefer fan-forced, the general rule is that the temperature is 20°C lower than the conventional temperatures given throughout the book. The cooking time may also be shorter—test for doneness a little earlier than the time advised. Personally, I'm happy sticking to conventional temperatures.

Washing fruit and vegetables—and this is a must. Fruits and whole vegetables will usually only need to be rinsed under cold running water and then dried well with a paper towel. Leafy green vegetables and herbs, especially if they have dirt between their leaves, need to be soaked in a bowl of cold water and any dirt teased out with your fingers, and then rinsed and dried (on a paper towel or clean tea towel, or spun in a salad spinner if you have one).

How to boil an egg—soft or hard? Place the egg straight from the refrigerator in cold water in a small saucepan over medium heat. Bring the water to simmering point and simmer for I minute for soft-boiled or 5–8 minutes for hard-boiled. Use a slotted spoon to lift the egg out; place hardboiled eggs in a bowl of cold water to prevent discolouring (if the water gets warm, change it).

How to cook fresh beetroot—you may prefer it to canned. Trim the leaves off a bunch of beetroot about 3cm (1 in) above the roots—don't trim the base as this will cause the beetroot to bleed. Wrap the beetroot in foil and place in a roasting pan. Bake at 180°C/350°F/Gas Mark 4 for 1–1½ hours, until tender. Cool and then peel, wearing rubber gloves to prevent staining your hands. Slip off the skins and trim off the roots, then slice or cut as liked.

Cooktops—what's the number for low, medium and high heat? If your cooktop numbers go from 1 to 9 a good guide is 2 to 4 for low, 5 to 6 medium and 7 to 8 for high. If you are bringing large quantities of water to the boil, go for 9. But, once again, it will depend on your stove—some elements get a lot hotter than others.

Clean up—unless you are head chef in a restaurant, it's part of cooking! Unless you want to be shown up as a total amateur, clean up as you go. Having a mess around you only makes the task more challenging and attracts sarcastic comments from others about your competence in the kitchen. Your food will taste that much better if you can enjoy it against a background of order rather than chaos.

Conquer the Kitchen & Shrink Your Belly

BELLY-BUSTING RECIPES

Breakfast of Champions — start the day as you want to continue   88

On-toast Specials — light meals in a hurry   93

DIY Lunches — at home or pack it up to go   98

Easy Roasts — who doesn't love a roast?   104

Barbecue Winners — the opportunity to shine as head chef   114

Meat and Three Veg — reinforcing the balanced meal   120

Man Salads — hearty and wholesome: more than a green leaf   125

One-pot Wonders — yippee, minimal washing up   131

Cupboard Hunt — quick and easy meals from the pantry   137

Sweets — a small selection to satisfy that sweet tooth   143

Favourite Flavours — to boost basic to fantastic   151

BREAKFAST OF CHAMPIONS
MIX

Start your day as you mean to continue ...

Raisin, cranberry and walnut grain-ola

Makes 8 x ¾ cup serves • 1371kJ (327 calories) per serve (with milk or yoghurt)

½ cup walnut pieces
½ cup raisins
½ cup dried cranberries
½ cup dried apricots, roughly chopped
2 cups traditional rolled oats
2 cups bran cereal
1 teaspoon cinnamon

◊ PREP & COOK

Roast the walnuts in a non-stick frying pan over a really low heat for about ten minutes, stirring them occasionally so they toast on both sides. Keep an eye on them so that they don't burn. You'll know when the nuts are done by their rich golden colour and the lovely warm nutty aroma. Remove the pan from the heat and let them cool.

Chop the walnuts, raisins and cranberries so they are all about the same size.

◊ MIX & STORE

Combine the walnuts, raisins, cranberries, apricots, oats, bran cereal and cinnamon in a large bowl and mix well.

Transfer to an airtight storage container and store it in the kitchen cupboard. It will keep for weeks—if it lasts that long.

◊ SERVE

Put ¾ cup mix in a cereal bowl with ½ cup low-fat milk and ½ cup low-fat yoghurt (natural or vanilla flavoured).

◊ TIPS

- *Sprinkle over a scoop of low-fat yogurt or ice cream as a topping.*
- *Keep some in your desk drawer at work for a snack.*

◊ OPTION

- *Mix 'n match your favourite dried fruits and nuts. Good combos are sultanas and pecans, currants and almonds, and prunes and hazelnuts.*

CEREAL

Turning an everyday brekkie into something special.

Bix, fruit and pecans

Serves 1 • 2106kJ (503 calories) per serve

◊ PREP

Hull the strawberries and slice. If the strawberries are straight from the fridge, place them in a microwave-safe bowl, cover and microwave for 5 seconds to warm them up—you don't want to stew them. This is entirely optional but will improve their flavour (and you can imagine they're picked straight from the garden).

◊ SERVE

Place the breakfast biscuits in a cereal bowl, add the milk and top with the strawberries, banana and pecans.

3 large strawberries
3 wheat or oat breakfast biscuits
1 cup low-fat milk
1 small banana or ½ a medium one, sliced
10 pecan halves, roughly chopped

◊ TIP
- *If you only use half a medium banana, put the other half in the freezer—it will be perfect for making a smoothie: just blend the frozen banana up with some milk, yoghurt and a sprinkle of nutmeg or cinnamon.*

◊ OPTION
- *You could use ½ cup fresh blueberries or raspberries instead of the strawberries, or thawed frozen berries.*

PORRIDGE

Perfect for cold mornings.

Oats with honey and rhubarb

Serves 2   •   1455kJ (348 calories) per serve

1 cup traditional rolled oats
2 cups low-fat milk
2 teaspoons honey
½ cup stewed rhubarb (see recipe, page 147)

◊ PREP & COOK

Put the oats and 1 cup cold water into a saucepan and set aside to soak for 5 minutes.

Place the saucepan over a medium heat. Add 1 cup milk to the oats and bring to the boil, stirring occasionally.

Reduce the heat to low and cook for 3–5 minutes, stirring occasionally, until the mixture is creamy.

Meanwhile, warm two bowls by filling with hot water and letting them stand for a few minutes. Pour out the water and wipe dry.

◊ SERVE

Spoon the porridge into the warmed bowls and swirl honey and rhubarb over the top. Serve with the remaining milk.

◊ TIPS

- *Stewed rhubarb is great to have in the fridge for a quick snack with yoghurt or to make a rhubarb crumble (see recipe, page 146). You can also buy tubs of stewed rhubarb in the supermarket. Save time making porridge in your microwave, following the directions on the back of the oats packet.*

◊ OPTIONS

- *Use ½ cup canned fruit, such as sour cherries or red plums, all available in natural juice instead of the stewed rhubarb—it's easy. Golden syrup or maple syrup is great instead of the honey.*

FRY

Enjoying a 'fry up' isn't a thing of the past. Tuck into this healthy one. The great thing about this recipe (besides the obvious) is you only use one large frying pan, and that means less washing up.

Bacon 'n' egg brekkie

Serves 1 • 1860kJ (444 calories) per serve

◊ PREP & COOK

Trim any visible fat off the bacon. Break the egg into a small bowl.

Heat a large non-stick frying pan over medium heat. When hot, add the oil and heat for a few seconds. Place the tomato halves, cut side down, along one side of the pan and the mushrooms on the other. Arrange the bacon centre stage right in the middle of the pan.

Cook the tomato and bacon for 2–3 minutes. Stir the mushrooms while cooking. Make a space in the pan around the side and slide in the egg, then turn the tomato and bacon and cook for 3 minutes.

Turn off the heat and cover the pan for about 1 minute, until the egg is cooked as liked.

Meanwhile, toast the muffin and spread with margarine.

◊ SERVE

Place the tomato, cut side up, on a warmed plate with the mushrooms and bacon. Slide out the egg using an egg lift and place it on top of the mushrooms and bacon. Scatter over the chives and serve the muffin on the side.

2 lean shortcut bacon rashers
1 egg
2 teaspoons oil
1 large tomato, halved across the middle
1 large flat mushroom, stalk trimmed and thickly sliced
1 multigrain muffin, split in half
2 teaspoons salt-reduced margarine spread
15 chives, snipped, for garnish

◊ TIP
- Using any fresh herbs adds great flavour.

◊ OPTION
- Leftover chunks of lean ham off the bone are great instead of bacon but don't be too heavy-handed with the amount. If you're an XL guy, you can have two eggs instead of one.

Belly-busting Recipes

MELT

If you close your eyes, you could be in Italy.

Tomato, basil, bean and two cheeses
Serves 1 • 1887kJ (451 calories) per serve

2 medium roma tomatoes
½ cup canned kidney beans, rinsed and drained
20 basil leaves, very finely shredded
2 tablespoons low-fat ricotta
2 slices wholemeal multigrain bread
2 teaspoons salt-reduced margarine spread
3 tablespoons finely grated parmesan cheese
freshly ground pepper

◊ PREP & COOK

Place a piece of foil on a grill tray and turn the grill to medium-to-high heat.

Slice the top and bottom off the tomatoes and cut each into four thick slices.

Put the kidney beans in a bowl and roughly mash with a fork. Mix in the basil and ricotta.

Toast the bread lightly under the grill and spread with the margarine.

Arrange the tomato on the toast and pile on the ricotta, bean and basil mixture. Sprinkle with the parmesan.

◊ GRILL

Place the melts on the grill tray and cook for about 5 minutes, until hot and the cheese is golden. Transfer the melts using an egg lift to a cutting board and cut as you like.

◊ SERVE

Leave the melts on the board or transfer them to a plate and sprinkle with pepper (or you could even wrap them and run).

◊ TIP
- *You need a sharp knife to slice tomatoes cleanly. You can buy a special tomato slicing knife.*

◊ OPTION
- *You could use low-fat cottage cheese instead of ricotta.*

ON-TOAST SPECIALS
EGGS

The perfect thing to make for your other half this Sunday morning.

Scrambled eggs with spinach, walnuts and feta

Serves 2 • 1881kJ (449 calories) per serve

◇ PREP & COOK

Break the eggs into a bowl and whisk lightly.

Roast the walnuts in a non-stick frying pan over low heat for about 10 minutes, stirring them occasionally. Keep an eye on them so that they don't burn. You'll know when the nuts are done by their rich golden colour and the lovely toasty aroma. Cool.

Wipe the pan out with a paper towel. Reduce the heat to low and put the pan back on the heat. Add the milk to the pan with 2 teaspoons of the margarine. When the milk is hot and the margarine has melted, stir in the egg. Gently lift and fold the egg—a kitchen spatula is good for this job—until the egg is set yet still creamy. Stir in the spinach leaves and cook until just wilted.

Toast the bread and spread with the remaining margarine.

◇ SERVE

Place the toast on warmed plates. Lift out the egg and spinach using the spatula and place it on the toast. Sprinkle over the walnuts, crumble the feta cheese on top and sprinkle with nutmeg.

◇ TIP
- *Baby rocket and pinenuts could be used instead of the spinach and walnuts.*

4 eggs
10 walnut halves
½ cup low-fat milk
1 tablespoon salt-reduced margarine spread
2 cups baby spinach leaves
2 slices wholegrain and oat bread
2 tablespoons low-fat feta cheese
¼–½ teaspoon ground nutmeg

TOMATOES

The depth of flavour of these tomatoes is amazing and their versatility is endless.

Sumac slow-roasted tomatoes with avocado

Serves 2 • 1660kJ (396 calories) per serve

3 medium roma tomatoes
4 cloves garlic, peeled
1 tablespoon sumac
1 teaspoon sugar
1 tablespoon oil
1 small avocado
4 slices wholemeal sourdough bread

◊ PREP & COOK

Preheat the oven to 180°C/350°F/Gas Mark 4. Line a small roasting pan with baking paper.

Cut the tomatoes in half lengthways. Put the tomatoes, cut side up, and garlic cloves in the roasting pan—they should fit snugly. Sprinkle with the sumac and sugar. Roast for 30 minutes, then lower the oven temperature to 120°C/250°F/Gas Mark 4 and roast for a further 1½ hours. Cool slightly.

◊ EXTRA PREP

Cut each piece of tomato in half lengthways and peel off their skins. Slice the garlic thinly. Cut the avocado in half and remove the seed. Toast the bread.

◊ SERVE

Place the toast on warmed plates. Scoop out the avocado flesh—a dessert spoon is good for this—and divide evenly between each slice of toast. Top the toast with the tomatoes and garlic.

◊ TIPS

- Sumac is a Middle Eastern red spice powder of crushed sumac berries. It has a tangy lemony taste and is a perfect match for tomatoes and avocado. You could use paprika instead.
- A stash of slow-roasted tomatoes made ahead is great to have in the fridge for this recipe or to toss though pasta, add to salads, sandwiches or wraps. Do yourself a favour and try the tomatoes with the Beetroot salad page 128.
- Always bring tomatoes to room temperature before eating to experience their full flavour (they are best not kept in the fridge).

MUSHROOMS

Mushrooms with style and a good kick start to a nice dinner.

Sherry and smoked paprika mushrooms

Serves 2 • 1400kJ (334 calories) per serve

◊ PREP & COOK

Trim the mushroom stalks and brush off any dirt—they don't need to be peeled or washed unless they are extremely dirty. Cut the small mushrooms into quarters and the flat mushroom into similar sized pieces.

Slice the roots and about one-third of the green tops off the spring onions and discard, then slice the remaining onion (but not too thinly); put the white part and the green part into separate bowls.

Heat the oil in a non-stick frying pan over medium heat. Add the sliced white onion and cook, stirring, for 1–2 minutes.

Add the mushrooms to the pan and cook until they soften, about 3 minutes, stirring occasionally. Sprinkle over the paprika and stir it in for about a minute. Add the beans next and keep giving the mixture a stir until everything is hot.

Pour over the sherry—it will sizzle and evaporate quickly—then toss in half of the green part of the spring onions.

Meanwhile, toast the bread.

◊ SERVE

Place the toast on warmed plates, spoon the mushrooms onto the toast and sprinkle with the remaining spring onion.

1 large flat mushroom
150g (5oz) small mushrooms
4 spring onions
1 tablespoon oil
2 teaspoons smoked paprika
½ cup canned cannellini beans, drained and rinsed
2 tablespoons medium dry sherry
4 slices soy and linseed bread

◊ TIPS
- *Smoked paprika is a red spice powder with a great smokey flavour. You can get it in supermarkets.*
- *Using Spanish smoked paprika and sherry make these mushrooms really amazing.*

◊ OPTION
- *You can use only one variety or a mixture of any mushrooms.*

SALMON

You could even serve this with a glass of bubbles for a special occasion brunch.

Salmon with lemon dill yoghurt

Serves 2 • 1461kJ (349 calories) per serve

4 sprigs dill, finely chopped
zest of 1 small lemon
½ cup plain low-fat yoghurt
2 Lebanese cucumbers
10 grape tomatoes
125g (4oz) can salmon slices
4 slices multigrain baguette

◊ PREP

Mix together the dill, lemon zest and yoghurt in a small bowl.
Top and tail the cucumbers and cut in half from the stalk. Scoop out the seeds of one of the cucumbers—the perfect tool for this job is a small teaspoon. (You could leave the seeds in if you like but removing them is worth the fuss.) Chop the cucumber flesh finely and stir into the lemon and dill yoghurt.
Cut the second cucumber into eight irregular chunks and place into a bowl with the tomatoes. Drain the salmon slices. Toast the bread.

◊ SERVE

Place the toast on plates and top with the lemon and dill yoghurt and the salmon slices. Place the cucumber chunks and tomatoes on the side.

◊ TIP
- *Fill two glasses with ice cubes, squeeze over the juice of the lemon and top with water. Add a sprig of mint and enjoy!*

◊ OPTION
- *You could use fresh or dried chives or dried dill instead of fresh.*
- *You could use smoked salmon instead of canned salmon.*

BEANS

These are so much better than the ones in a can.

DIY baked beans

Serves 2 • 1827kJ (436 calories) per serve

◊ PREP & COOK

Trim any excess fat off the bacon and chop the bacon finely. Heat the oil in a non-stick saucepan over a medium high heat. Add the bacon and, stirring occasionally, cook until it starts to brown, 2–3 minutes.

Turn the heat to low, stir in the onion and cook for 3–5 minutes, until it softens. Add the tomato paste, tomatoes and Worcestershire sauce and keep stirring until the mixture comes to the boil.

Add the cannellini beans and simmer, stirring occasionally, for 5 minutes.

Meanwhile, split the muffins in half and toast them.

◊ SERVE

Place the toasted muffins on warmed plates and pile the beans on top.

◊ TIPS

- *Chopped coriander or parsley leaves give another dimension to the beans when sprinkled on top.*
- *If you like it hot, sprinkle over some chilli flakes or sauce.*

◊ OPTION

- *You can cook up dried cannellini beans instead of using canned beans—they are more economical and can be frozen in meal-size containers until you need them. Simply soak the beans in water overnight, then discard the water the next day. Place them in a large pan with plenty of water and bring to the boil (don't add any salt or they will take ages to cook—and you are better off shaking the salt habit.) Simmer for around an hour, until they're soft.*

2 lean rashers streaky bacon
1 tablespoon oil
1 medium red onion, sliced
2 tablespoons tomato paste (with no added salt)
400g (14oz) can whole tomatoes
2 teaspoons Worcestershire sauce
410g (14½oz) can cannellini beans, rinsed and drained
2 multigrain muffins

DIY LUNCHES
ROLL

Feed the man beef, but make it tasty and keep it lean.

Mustard and horseradish beef salad

Serves 1 • 1830kJ (437 calories) per serve

1 large wholegrain bread roll, cut in half

2 teaspoons salt-reduced margarine spread

2 teaspoons wholegrain mustard

2 teaspoons horseradish cream

80g (2½oz) shaved lean rare roast beef

½ small red pepper, sliced

1 small Lebanese cucumber, sliced

½ cup mixed lettuce leaves

◊ PREP

Get everything out on the bench ready before you start.

◊ MAKE

Spread each half of the roll with margarine, then spread one half with the mustard and the other with horseradish cream.

Layer the bottom half with the beef, red pepper, cucumber and lettuce and place the other half roll on top.

Cut as you prefer or wrap your man-hands around the whole thing and devour.

◊ SERVE OR PACK

Put the filled roll on a plate to eat immediately. Alternatively, wrap it to go in baking paper and a brown paper bag; keep the roll cold in a cooler bag if making it to go.

◊ TIP
- *Leftover beef from the previous night's roast is delicious in this recipe (see beef recipe, page 107).*

◊ OPTION
- *Use shaved chicken instead of the beef.*

WRAP

You'll be wrapped with this wrap.

Egg, dukkah mayonnaise and rocket wrap

Serves 1 • 1687kJ (403 calories) per serve

◊ PREP & COOK

Place the eggs, if they come straight from the fridge, in a saucepan of cold water over a medium heat. (Eggs at room temperature may be placed straight into boiling water.) Bring to the boil, reduce heat and simmer 8–10 minutes. Drain. Cover the eggs with cold water, replacing the water if it gets warm. When the eggs are cold, remove the shell and slice.

Make the dukkah mayonnaise by mixing the yoghurt, mayonnaise and dukkah in a small bowl.

◊ MAKE

Lay the cornbread on a piece of baking paper that's larger than the bread. Arrange the rocket, carrot and egg over the bread. Drizzle with the dukkah mayonnaise. Roll up tightly in the baking paper, twisting the ends of the paper to close.

◊ SERVE

Cut the wrap in half diagonally and eat by rolling back the paper.

2 eggs
2 tablespoons low-fat natural yoghurt
1 tablespoon mayonnaise
2 teaspoons dukkah
1 piece flat cornbread or lavash
¼ cup baby rocket
1 small carrot, grated

◊ WHAT IS …
- *Dukkah is a Middle Eastern blend of roasted nuts and seeds and is available in specialty herb and spice shops and delicatessens. Or make your own dukkah (see recipe, page 152).*

◊ OPTION
- *Love curried eggs? Easy. Use 1–2 teaspoons of your favourite curry powder instead of the dukkah.*

NOODLES

Thank goodness for the great food that comes from Asia.

Tuna, sweet soy, lemon ginger dressing

Serves 1 • 1911kJ (456 calories) per serve

65g (2oz) dry rice vermicelli noodles
2cm (¾in) piece of ginger, peeled and grated
3 teaspoons kecap manis (sweet soy sauce)
1 teaspoon lemon juice
2 teaspoons sesame oil
4 spring onions, trimmed and chopped
1 small red pepper, roughly chopped
125g (4oz) can tuna slices in spring water, drained

◊ WHAT IS ...

Kecap manis (pronounced kechap maniss) is a sweet soy sauce used in Indonesian and Malaysian cuisine. You'll find it with the Asian sauces in the supermarket.

◊ PREP

Place the noodles in a bowl and cover with boiling water. Stand for about 3 minutes until soft. Rinse, drain well and put into a dry bowl (if you leave them wet, the dressing won't stick).

Make the dressing by mixing together the ginger, kecap manis, lemon juice, and sesame oil (see Tip) in a small bowl.

◊ MAKE

Stir the spring onions, red pepper and tuna into the noodles and drizzle over the dressing.

◊ SERVE OR PACK

Eat straight out of the bowl or pack in a container for later. The flavour will develop even more overnight in the fridge. For a work lunch keep it cold in an insulated bag with an ice brick.

◊ TIPS

- Add the sesame oil just before eating for a more intense flavour.
- Try adding a handful of finely chopped coriander or mint as well.

◊ OPTIONS

- Double, triple or quadruple the recipe to feed two, three or four people.
- You could use instant noodles but make sure they're low fat.

PASTA

This is a great way to use up leftovers such as pasta and our Studded rosemary & garlic leg of lamb (see recipe, page 104).

Lamb and pesto penne

Serves 1 • 2505kJ (598 calories) per serve

◊ PREP

Make the pesto by placing the basil leaves, parmesan, pinenuts and olive oil into the bowl of a small food processor and process for 1–2 minutes until well mixed. If you don't have a food processor you can use a mortar and pestle.

◊ MAKE

Put the pasta in a bowl, stir in the pesto, lamb, tomatoes and olives.

◊ SERVE OR PACK

Eat out of the bowl now or pack in a container for later. Keep it cold in the fridge or carry it in an insulated bag with an ice brick.

½ cup loosely packed basil leaves

10g (⅓oz) piece of parmesan cheese, roughly chopped (see tip)

1 tablespoon pinenuts

2 teaspoons extra virgin olive oil

1 cup cooked penne pasta

80g (2½oz) sliced lean (no white stuff) roast lamb

8 small cherry tomatoes

5 small pitted kalamata olives

◊ TIPS

- If you don't have any leftover penne, here's how to cook it. Fill a small pot about three-quarters full with water and bring to the boil. Add the penne and cook, uncovered, for about 11 minutes. Test that the penne is cooked by tasting. The Italians say it should be 'al dente', or firm rather than soft.
- You could use 2 tablespoons of finely grated parmesan instead of the chopped cheese.
- Use prepared pesto from the delicatessen or supermarket if you prefer.

◊ OPTION

- Use your favourite pasta shapes.

RICE

Chicken and rice just got a whole lot more interesting.

Tandoori chicken rice

Serves 1 • 2054kJ (491 calories) per serve

Ingredients:

- 1 chicken breast
- 1 tablespoon low-fat natural yoghurt
- 1 tablespoon tandoori paste
- ¼ cup basmati or low-GI rice
- spray oil
- 1 small Lebanese cucumber, finely chopped
- 1 medium tomato, finely chopped
- 20 fresh mint leaves

◊ PREP

Trim any fat from the chicken breast. Make 3–4 evenly spaced cuts (but not all the way through) in the top of the breast using a sharp pointed knife.

Mix 2 teaspoons of yoghurt with the tandoori paste.

Place the chicken on a plate and coat each side with the yoghurt. Cover the chicken with plastic wrap and refrigerate for at least two hours.

◊ COOK & MAKE

Place the rice in a small saucepan and cover with ¾ cup of cold water. Bring to the boil over medium heat, stirring constantly. Reduce the heat to low, cover, and cook without stirring for 8–10 minutes. Stir the rice and cool.

Heat a small non-stick frying pan over a low-to-medium heat. When hot, spray with the oil. Place the chicken in the pan and cook for 4 minutes, turn chicken and cook for a further 3 minutes or until cooked through (take care— it may spit). Wrap the chicken in foil and rest for 5 minutes.

Stir the cucumber, tomato and mint into the rice.

Slice the chicken thinly and add to the rice along with any cooking juices.

◊ SERVE

Place in a bowl to eat immediately or pack in a container for later. Keep it cold in the fridge until you leave and carry in a cooler bag with an ice brick.

◊ TIPS

- *Cook the chicken in the oven, on a grill or barbecue if you prefer.*

- Check the cooking instructions on the rice pack. They usually give you several options—try them all and see which you like best.
  ◊ OPTIONS
- You can use pre-cooked rice—either leftovers or in packets called '90-second rice' (get the brown one for extra goodness).
- Tandoori paste is available in supermarkets—once opened keep it in the fridge.

EASY ROASTS
LAMB

Since you're turning on the oven, why not go the whole hog and roast some vegetables too?

Studded rosemary and garlic leg of lamb

Serves 8 • 1069kJ (255 calories) per serve

1.5kg (3lb 5oz) lean leg of lamb on the bone
12 sprigs rosemary
4 cloves garlic, peeled
1 cup reduced-salt beef stock

◊ PREP

Preheat the oven to 180°C/350°F/Gas Mark 4.

Trim any visible fat from the leg of lamb. Use a sharp pointed knife to make 12 evenly spaced incisions in the lamb. Cut each clove of garlic lengthways into three pieces. Push a sprig of rosemary and a piece of garlic into each of the cuts on the lamb.

Place the leg of lamb on a rack in a roasting pan. Pour the stock into the bottom of the roasting pan.

◊ COOK

Place the roasting pan in the middle of the oven. Cook the lamb for 1 hour for rare, 1¼ hours for medium or 1½ hours for well done (see Tip).

Transfer the roasted lamb to a large plate or tray and discard the stock. Cover the meat loosely with foil and allow it to rest for about 15 minutes.

◊ SERVE

Carve the lamb as thinly or thickly sliced as liked—it's great and rustic just chopped into chunks too.

Serve on warmed plates the traditional way with roasted vegetables (see recipe, page 113) and mint sauce (see recipe, page 158). It's OK to serve with bought mint sauce (or mint jelly)—there are some great ones around.

◊ TIPS

- *Cold leftover lamb has lots of uses—see the Lamb and pesto penne (recipe, page 101), on sandwiches or even in a quick curry.*
- *You could cook in a barbecue with a lid.*

- For a juicy and succulent result, cook the leg either rare or medium.
- Using a meat thermometer helps to cook the meat to perfection—place the thermometer in the thickest part of the lamb. The internal temperature of the meat for a rare leg will be 55–60°C (130–140°F), medium 65–70°C (150–160°F) or for well done 75°C (165°F).

◇ OPTION

- For a Mediterranean twist, serve with a Tossed salad (see recipe, page 125) and Tzatziki (see recipe, page 154) and lots of lemon wedges.

FISH 'N CHIPS

Here's a 'better for you' version of a perennial favourite.

Salmon, chips and salad

Serves 2 • 2679kJ (640 calories) per serve

2 x 200g (7oz) skinless, pin-boned salmon fillet, 2cm (¾in) thick

500g (1lb 2oz) waxy potatoes

2 tablespoons sweet chilli sauce

1 tablespoon lime juice

2 teaspoons kecap manis

2 tablespoons oil

¼ small iceberg lettuce, cut into two even wedges

12 cherry tomatoes, quartered

8 large basil leaves, cut into very fine shreds

◇ OPTION
- Ask your fishmonger about what's best on the day—you can use any fresh fish fillets.

◇ WHAT IS …

'Pin-boned' means extracting any bones with a pair of kitchen tweezers.

◇ PREP

Preheat the oven to 200°C/400°F/Gas Mark 6. Take the fish out of the fridge, keep it covered and bring it to room temperature before cooking. Cut the potatoes into chips about 10 x 3cm (4 x 1¼in). Pat them dry with a paper towel.

Make the dressing by mixing the sweet chilli sauce, lime juice and kecap manis in a small bowl. Take out about a teaspoon of this mixture to use as the glaze.

◇ COOK

Heat a roasting pan in the hot oven. Toss the chips and oil in a bowl, coating evenly. Arrange the chips in a single layer in the hot roasting pan and drizzle over any remaining oil. Roast for 15 minutes before turning and cooking for a further 10 minutes.

Make room in the pan for the fish by pushing the chips towards the edges, still keeping them in a single layer. Place the fish in the pan and cook for 2 minutes. Turn the fish, brush the top with the glaze and cook for 2 minutes longer—the fish needs to still be pinky red in the centre.

Transfer the fish to a warm plate and cover loosely with foil.

Test that the chips are done by inserting a skewer into a couple—they should be firm but cooked through (you could cool one and do a taste test to make sure they are done to your liking).

◇ SERVE

Divide the fish, chips and lettuce between two plates. Top the fish with the tomatoes and basil and drizzle over the dressing.

◇ TIP
- Always discard any uncooked glaze or marinade that has been used on raw food (it has bacteria).

BEEF

This little piggy had roast beef ... and thoroughly enjoyed it!

Succulent roast beef

Serves 4 • 1550kJ (370 calories) per serve

◊ PREP

Preheat the oven to 220°C/420°F/Gas Mark 7.

Trim any visible fat from the beef and place on a rack in a roasting pan. Pour the stock into the bottom of the roasting pan.

◊ COOK

Place the roasting pan in the middle of the oven. Cook the beef for 10 minutes, then reduce the temperature to 200°C (400°F) and cook for a further 15–20 minutes for medium rare (if using a meat thermometer, see Tips).

Transfer the beef to a large tray or plate, cover loosely with foil and rest the meat for 20 minutes. Discard the stock.

◊ SERVE

Carve the beef very finely—almost shaved is best—and serve in warmed bowls with the Roasted capsicum with onions and garlic (see recipe, page 112) and the horseradish cream. Use the bread to soak up the juices.

800g (1lb 13oz) piece lean boneless topside
1 cup reduced-salt beef stock
2 tablespoons horseradish cream to serve
2 long wholemeal bread rolls, sliced, to serve

◊ TIPS
- If using a meat thermometer, the internal temperature will be 65–70°C (150–160°F). If you prefer the meat rare, it will only need 10–15 minutes extra (not 15–20) and the internal temperature will be 55–60°C (130–140°F). For well done, roast the meat for 25–30 minutes at 200°C (400°F); the internal temperature needs to reach 75°C (165°F).
- Sharpen your knife to carve really thin slices.
- Allow resting time for the juices to redistribute for juicy, succulent, tasty beef.
- Follow the same temperatures and cooking times for beef fillet or scotch fillet.

◊ OPTIONS
- Serve the beef with Dijon or wholegrain mustard or redcurrant jelly instead of horseradish cream.
- Make leftover beef into lunch wraps or sandwiches with salad.

CHICKEN

Those Moroccans sure know what they're doing with poultry.

Spiced Moroccan chicken with lemon

Serves 2, plus leftovers • 1443kJ (345 calories) per serve (chicken and yoghurt only)

1.5kg (3lb 5oz) chicken
1 lemon, halved
1 teaspoon ground cumin
1 teaspoon ground coriander
¼ teaspoon paprika
¼ teaspoon ground cinnamon
1 tablespoon oil
1 cup salt-reduced chicken stock
Cumin potatoes, carrot and bean couscous (see recipe, page 110)
2 tablespoons low-fat natural yoghurt

◊ PREP

Preheat the oven to 180°C/350°F/Gas Mark 4.

Remove any visible fat from the chicken and discard—check the cavity as well. Rinse and thoroughly dry the chicken inside and out with a paper towel.

Place the chicken, breast side up, on a rack in a roasting pan, squeeze over lemon juice then put the squeezed lemon halves into the cavity.

Make the spice blend by mixing together the ground cumin, coriander, paprika and cinnamon in a small bowl.

Work your fingers under the skin of the chicken to loosen it (take care not to tear it) and massage about three-quarters of the spice mix into the meat under the skin. Mix the remaining spice mix with a teaspoon of the oil and rub over the outside of the chicken. Tie the legs together with a piece of kitchen string.

Pour the stock into the bottom of a roasting pan, put a rack on top and place the chicken on the rack.

◊ COOK

Put the roasting pan in the middle of the heated oven. Roast the chicken for 1¼ hours—about 25 minutes per 500g/1lb.

Meanwhile, make the couscous—it's good economy to cook it with the chicken.

Test if the chicken is cooked by inserting a skewer into the thickest part of the leg—if the juices run clear it is cooked.

Transfer the chicken to a large tray or plate, cover loosely with foil and rest it for 10–15 minutes. Discard the stock.

◊ SERVE

Carve the breast portions from the chicken and remove the wings. Cover the rest of the bird (see Tips).

Place the breasts on warmed plates, spoon over some yoghurt and serve with Cumin potatoes, carrot and beans couscous.

◊ TIPS
- *Strip the meat from the remaining chicken. Use the meat in salads and sandwiches or freeze for another time. This is perfect for a quick curry or stew.*
- *The bones and skin could be cooked up for stock—you'll need to refrigerate the stock overnight and remove any hard white fat that settles on top.*

COUSCOUS

The Moroccan magic continues—put the veggies in the oven while your chicken is roasting.

Cumin potatoes, carrot and bean couscous

Serves 2 • 1697kJ (405 calories) per serve

250g (9oz) waxy potatoes (about 2)
2 medium carrots, peeled
100g (3½oz) beans
1 tablespoon oil
2 teaspoons cumin seeds
½ cup couscous
2 teaspoons salt-reduced margarine spread

◊ PREP

Preheat the oven to 180°C/350°F/Gas Mark 4 (cook with the chicken if serving with the Spiced Moroccan chicken and lemon (see recipe, page 108).

Wash and dry the potatoes. Cut each potato into quarters lengthways—they'll be about 5 x 5cm (2 x 2in). Pat them dry with a paper towel. Slice the carrots into large 3cm (1¼in) chunks. Top and tail the beans and cut in half.

Place the potatoes and carrot in a roasting pan, add the oil and toss until the vegetables are well coated. Sprinkle over the cumin seeds.

◊ COOK

Roast the vegetables in the middle shelf of the oven for about 30 minutes, until they are firm but cooked through—insert a skewer into the centre of a few to test.

Meanwhile, bring a small amount of water in a saucepan to the boil over a medium heat. Add the beans and cook for 2–3 minutes, until they turn bright green, drain (see Tip).

To cook the couscous, bring ½ cup water to the boil over medium heat. Remove from the heat and stir in the couscous, cover, and stand for 2–3 minutes. Stir in the margarine. Break up the grains with a fork and stir into the vegetables with the beans.

◊ SERVE

Serve with Spiced Moroccan and lemon chicken, beef or lamb roasts and anything barbecued.

◊ TIPS

- Eat hot or cold and add some fresh herbs and a dollop of low-fat natural yoghurt.

- Cook the couscous on the bottom shelf of the oven at the same time as cooking a roast—allow more time if sharing the oven and remember it can keep cooking while the roast is resting.
- You can also microwave the beans for 1½ minutes on high (no water is needed)

◊ OPTIONS
- You could substitute sweet potato or pumpkin for carrot.
- Courgettes, squash or asparagus could be used instead of beans.

◊ WHAT IS ...
Couscous is the ground starchy part of durum wheat (semolina) and is miraculously fast to prepare—just add hot water or stock (and whatever spices you like). It's actually a type of pasta.

PEPPERS

These roasted vegetables have incredible flavour.

Roasted peppers with onions and garlic

Serves 4 • 603kJ (144 calories) per serve

2 medium red peppers
2 medium brown onions, unpeeled
1 whole head of garlic, unpeeled
1 tablespoon oil
10 mini roma tomatoes, halved
2 teaspoons ground cumin
2 cups frozen peas
2 tablespoons finely shredded mint

◊ TIPS
- If cooking this at the same as the Succulent roast beef, place the vegetables on the bottom shelf—reduce their cooking time by 5-10 minutes as they will cook faster in the hotter oven.
- You could microwave the peas for 3-4 minutes on high—no need to add water.

◊ PREP

Preheat the oven to 180°C/350°F/Gas Mark 4.

Wash the peppers and dry well. Trim the roots and brush off any dirt around the roots of the onion and garlic.

Place the whole peppers and unpeeled onions and garlic in a roasting pan and brush with oil.

◊ COOK

Roast the vegetables in the middle shelf of the oven (see Tips) for about 40 minutes, until the peppers are soft. Transfer the peppers and garlic to a bowl. Continue roasting the onions for another 20 minutes.

Peel the skin off the peppers once they have cooled enough to be handled. Break the flesh into pieces and put in another bowl with any juices; discard the skins and seeds. Cut the top off the garlic and squeeze out the garlic paste into the peppers.

When the onions are cool enough to handle, peel off their skins. Cut the onions into large wedges. Add to the peppers and garlic.

Stir in the tomatoes—the residual heat from the roasted vegetables will warm them up—and the cumin.

Meanwhile, bring a small amount of water to the boil over a medium heat (see Tips). Add the peas and cook 2–3 minutes, until they turn bright green. Drain and stir into the peppers.

◊ SERVE

Hot or at room temperature sprinkled with mint with Succulent roast beef (see recipe, page 107) or any roast or barbecued meats.

POTATOES

These traditional roast vegetables will warm the cockles of your heart

Traditional potatoes roasted with pumpkin

Serves 4 • 1015kJ (242 calories) per serve

◊ PREP

Preheat the oven to 180°C/350°F/Gas Mark 4.

Cut each potato in half or thirds, depending on the size. Pat dry with a paper towel. Cut the sweet potato and pumpkin into similar-sized pieces and dry with a paper towel.

Put the potato, sweet potato, pumpkin, onion and tomato into a roasting pan and brush them well with oil.

◊ COOK

Roast the vegetables in the middle shelf of the oven for 30–40 minutes, turning them once, until they are golden and tender.

◊ SERVE

Serve the vegetables immediately with the Studded rosemary and garlic leg of lamb (see recipe, page 104), peas, Mint sauce (page 158) and Gravy (page 157) for a traditional roast meal or with any roasted meats.

500g (1lb 2oz) waxy potatoes (about 4)
1 large gold sweet potato, peeled
500g (1lb 2oz) butternut pumpkin, peeled and de-seeded
1 tablespoon oil
2 brown onions, peeled and halved
2 medium tomatoes, halved

◊ TIPS

- *It is important to dry foods well before roasting to ensure they go crisp and not soggy.*
- *Turn up the oven towards the end of the cooking time if you prefer really golden, crisp vegetables.*
- *If you're doing these with roast meat, give them a blast of heat on the bottom shelf while the roast is resting.*

◊ OPTION

- *Pumpkin, parsnip, garlic, courgettes, squash and aubergines can all be roasted instead of these traditional vegetables.*

BARBECUE WINNERS
STEAK

Every man needs to perfect the art of the steak. Buy the best quality steak you can afford—go for quality not quantity. Choose thick steaks rather than thin—this prevents overcooking, whether you prefer a rare or medium rare steak.

The perfect barbecue steak

Serves 4 • 1245kJ (297 calories) per serve

2 x 200g (7oz) beef fillets or rump steaks
¼–½ teaspoon oil per steak

◊ PREP

Take the steak out of the fridge early, keep it covered and bring to room temperature. Make sure any salads you are serving are ready before you start cooking.

Fire up the barbecue—it needs to be really hot to brown and caramelise the meat.

Trim any visible fat off the steaks. Rub or brush the oil on the steaks—don't oil the barbecue grill or hotplate.

◊ COOK

Place the steaks on the hot barbecue (the grill part is better than the hotplate for steaks). Resist the temptation to turn the meat—it only needs to be turned once during cooking.

Turn the steak when the first sign of moisture appears on the upper side and cook as you like. Press tongs on the meat to test the doneness of the steak—rare is soft, medium is springy and well done is firm.

Rest the meat by transferring it to a clean plate and covering it loosely with foil. Resting for about 5 minutes will ensure that the steak is really juicy. This is because the juices, which had gone to the centre of the meat during cooking, will be redistributed.

◊ SERVE

Place on individual plates and pour the delicious juices over each steak. Serve with the Spuds and Tossed salad (pages 126 and 125).

◊ TIPS
- Choose 1cm (½in) thick steaks for well-done steak lovers and about 3cm (1¼in) thick steaks for those who prefer rare—this helps even up the cooking times when cooking for a crowd.
- Corn cobs are always a great hit at barbecues—cook up a few—you can keep turning these as much as you like so they are browned all over. It's a great thing to do while catching up with mates over a (light) cool ale. Serve the corn as a starter or with the meat and salad.
- The Beetroot salad (page 128) would also be great for a crowd.

◊ OPTION
- Sizzle some lamb rump steaks for a change.

STEAK AND PRAWNS

A man needs to master the classics.

Steak, prawns and aioli

Serves 2 • 1975kJ (472 calories) per serve (without bread salad)

8 green king prawns, unpeeled
2 bunches asparagus
2 x 200g (7oz) beef fillet steaks
1–2 teaspoons oil
1 tablespoon Aioli (garlic mayonnaise; see recipe, page 155)
Bread salad (see recipe, page 129)

◊ PREP

Fire up the barbecue.

Shell and devein the prawns but leave their tails on. To devein prawns, make a shallow cut along the back to expose the dark-coloured gut and remove it.

Snap off the woody ends of the asparagus spears and cut a cross into the base of each spear—this helps the spears to cook evenly.

Trim any visible fat off the steaks. Rub half the oil on the steaks.

◊ COOK

Place the steak on the heated barbecue and cook to your taste (see page 115 for cooking tips). Rest the steaks for 5 minutes.

Meanwhile, heat the remaining oil on the barbecue and toss on the prawns and asparagus spears. Turn the prawns and asparagus once; the prawns will only take 1–2 minutes and, depending on their size, the asparagus needs about the same amount of time. The asparagus is cooked when the spears turn bright green.

◊ SERVE

Place the steak on warmed plates, top with the prawns and arrange the asparagus alongside.

Spoon the Aioli on top or serve separately and place the Bread salad centre stage in the middle of the table to share.

◊ OPTION
- Make the dish with fish fillets and prawns—as always with seafood, the fresher the better.

◊ TIP
- Use plain toasted bread in the Bread salad instead of the Olive and garlic bread if you feel a double hit of garlic from both the salad and aioli is a bit much!

Belly-busting Recipes

BURGERS

Tuck into this very civilised topless burger with a knife and fork.

Open beef burger with egg
Serves 2 • 2410kJ (576 calories) per serve

◊ PREP

Make the patties by mixing the mince, crumbs, parsley, Worcestershire sauce and one of the eggs (lightly beaten) in a bowl—using clean hands is easiest. Shape the mixture into two even-sized patties about 1cm (½in) thick. Place on a plate, cover and rest in the refrigerator for about 30 minutes.

Fire up the barbecue.

Spray the patties and the heated barbecue hotplate with oil.

◊ COOK

Cook the patties on the hotplate for about 4–5 minutes each side, turning once.

Meanwhile, fry the onions until golden and the extra two eggs as liked—egg rings are great for keeping the eggs in good shape (spray the inside of the rings with oil so the eggs slide out easily). Toast the bread.

◊ SERVE

Place the toast on warmed plates and top each with lettuce, a beef pattie, some onion, tomato slices, beetroot slices, pineapple, an egg and barbecue sauce.

◊ TIP
- There's no need to take the crust off the bread for the crumbs; one slice of bread will give you roughly ⅔ cup of soft breadcrumbs.
- Choose the best quality lean mince that you can afford.

◊ OPTIONS
- Use iceberg lettuce for a real retro burger experience.
- Add chopped coriander instead of parsley to the burger and eat with sweet chilli sauce for an Asian twist.

300g (10½oz) lean beef mince

breadcrumbs made from 1 slice day-old wholegrain and oats bread

2 tablespoons chopped parsley

1 teaspoon Worcestershire sauce

3 eggs

spray oil

1 large brown onion, sliced

2 slices wholegrain and oats bread

¼ cup lettuce leaves

1 large tomato, sliced

4 slices canned beetroot

2 slices canned pineapple

2 tablespoons barbecue sauce

KEBABS

Kebab is a Persian word for grilled meat.

Honey mustard glazed pork kebabs
Serves 2 • 1916kJ (458 calories) per serve

4 long bamboo skewers
2 tablespoons honey
1 teaspoon Dijon mustard
2 teaspoons barbecue sauce
400g (14oz) lean pork leg steak
1 small red pepper
1 small green pepper
16 small button mushrooms, stems trimmed
1 tablespoon oil

◊ PREP

Soak the bamboo skewers in water for 30 minutes.

Make the glaze by mixing together the honey, mustard and barbecue sauce in a small bowl. Cover and place in the fridge.

Cut the pork into 16 even-sized cubes (about 2cm/¾in) and the peppers into similar-sized pieces.

Thread the pork, peppers and mushrooms onto the skewers—starting and finishing with peppers works well and looks colourful.

Fire up the barbecue—these kebabs look great cooked on the grill section.

◊ COOK

Brush one side of the kebabs with oil and place on the barbecue, oil side down. Cook for about 5 minutes, then brush the tops with oil and turn. Cook for another 5 minutes or until cooked as you like.

Place the kebabs on a big piece of foil, brush all over with the glaze, wrap and rest for 5 minutes.

◊ SERVE

Place kebabs with their juices on warmed plates and serve with the Beetroot salad (page 128).

◊ TIP

- Save time and make the Beetroot salad without the garlic chips.

◊ WHAT IS ...

Pomegranate molasses is pomegranate concentrate and you'll find it in some supermarkets, Middle Eastern delicatessens and specialty food stores.

◊ OPTIONS

- Make a quick salad with leftover cooked brown rice and bits of pepper, fresh mint and salad dressing (see recipe, page 156—it's perfect to serve with the kebabs).
- Instead of honey, make the glaze with pomegranate molasses, which is delicious.

KOFTAS

Kofta is a Middle Eastern word for meatball or meatloaf.

Lamb in pita with tabouli and yoghurt

Serves 2 • 2919kJ (697 calories) per serve

◊ PREP

Soak the bamboo skewers in water for 30 minutes.

Make the koftas by mixing the mince, garlic, tomato, pomegranate molasses and spice in a bowl with clean hands. Shape the mixture onto the skewers, shaping it around the stick into a sausage shape.

Fire up the barbecue—the grill is best.

◊ COOK

Brush one side of the koftas with oil and place on the grill, oil side down. Grill for about 5 minutes, then brush the tops with oil and turn. Cook for another 5 minutes or until cooked.

Place the koftas on a baking tray, remove the sticks, cover with foil and keep warm.

◊ SERVE

Place the pita bread on warmed plates and top each piece with a scoop of tabouli, a kofta and a dollop of yoghurt.

◊ TIPS

- *Warm the pita bread on the barbecue if you prefer it heated.*
- *Make into wraps if it's a stand-up event. Wrap each firmly in a large piece of baking paper, twisting one end tightly.*
- *Baharat spice blend is available in delicatessens or online from specialty spice shops. Alternatively, you could make your own—see recipe, page 153.*

◊ OPTIONS

- *If you don't have pomegranate molasses, honey, golden or maple syrup make great substitutes.*
- *You could use lean beef or chicken mince to make the koftas.*
- *Make the mixture into small meatballs and fry in a little oil in a non-stick pan—they are great for dipping into Tzatziki.*

4 long bamboo skewers
400g (14oz) lean lamb mince
4 cloves garlic, peeled and crushed
2 small tomatoes, diced
2 teaspoons pomegranate molasses
2 tablespoons Baharat spice blend (see Tip)
2 teaspoons oil
2 x 75g (2½oz) medium-sized wholemeal flat breads, cut in half
½ quantity Tabouli (see recipe, page 130)
½ cup low-fat natural yoghurt

MEAT & THREE VEG
CUTLETS

Handy how Mother Nature made this lamb with handles.

Lamb cutlets and eggplant dip

Serves 2 • 2480kJ (592 calories) per serve

- 400g (14oz) rack lean lamb cutlets (8 cutlets)
- 2 medium courgettes, trimmed
- 2 medium tomatoes, halved
- 2 medium mushrooms, trimmed
- 1 tablespoon oil
- 250g (9oz) brown 90-second microwave rice
- 4 tablespoons aubergine dip (baba ghanoush), ready-made

◊ PREP

Turn the oven grill on to 180°C/350°F/Gas Mark 4. Adjust the grill tray to allow 5cm (2in) between the top of the meat and the heat.

Trim any visible fat from the rack of lamb and cut into 4 double cutlets (or ask the butcher to do this for you).

Cut the courgettes in half, lengthways.

Brush the skin side of the courgettes, tomatoes and mushrooms lightly with oil and one side of the cutlets.

◊ COOK

Place the cutlets, courgettes, tomato and mushrooms, oiled sides down, on the grill rack. Brush the tops of the vegetables and the cutlets with the remaining oil.

Grill for 5 minutes and then turn the cutlets—there's no need to turn the vegetables—and grill for a further 3–5 minutes, until the lamb is cooked as you like.

Place the lamb on a warm plate, cover with foil and rest for 5 minutes. If the vegetables are cooked—soft but still keeping their shape and lightly browned—turn off the grill and leave them to sit there while the lamb is resting; otherwise cook them for a little longer.

Meanwhile, microwave the rice following the manufacturer's directions.

◊ SERVE

Serve the rice, vegetables and cutlets with the aubergine dip over the cutlets.

◊ TIPS

- *The oven grill tray doesn't need to be right at the very top of the oven.*

- *If you prefer, you could cook on the grill of your barbecue or a grill pan on the top of the stove.*
  ◊ OPTIONS
- *Small finger aubergine could be used instead of courgettes and natural low-fat yoghurt mixed with chopped mint or coriander instead of the aubergine dip.*

MEATLOAF

Just like the album *Bat Out of Hell*, this meatloaf is an absolute classic with a surprise spicy note.

Beef and lentil meatloaf

Serves 2 with 1 serve meatloaf left over • 2359kJ (563 calories) per serve

½ cup red lentils
2 slices wholegrain and oats bread, torn up roughly
1 medium brown onion, peeled and chopped roughly
1 medium carrot, peeled and chopped roughly
½ cup tightly packed parsley leaves
400g (14oz) lean beef mince
2 tablespoons garam masala spice
1 egg, lightly beaten
3 tablespoons tomato chutney
2 cups loosely packed mixed lettuce leaves
olive oil, vinegar and herbs (see Salad dressing recipe, page 156)

◊ PREP

Preheat the oven to 180°C/350°F/Gas Mark 4.

Check the lentils for unwanted stones. Cover the lentils with water in a small saucepan, cover, and bring to the boil over a medium heat. Take off the lid and cook until the lentils have absorbed the water, 2–3 minutes. Cool.

Line a 7cm (2¾in) deep, 11 x 21cm (4½ x 8½in) loaf pan with a double layer of baking paper, bringing the paper up about 2cm (¾in) above the top of the pan—this will make it easy to remove the meatloaf.

Crumb the bread in a food processor, pulsing 5–6 times until crumbed. Add the onion, carrot and parsley to the crumbs and process for a further 2–3 minutes. Transfer the mixture to a large bowl. Add the lentils, mince, garam masala and egg.

Mix well with clean hands until well combined. Press the mixture into the prepared pan, pressing it down firmly until the top is smooth.

◊ COOK

Place the pan on the middle shelf of the oven and bake for 30–35 minutes, until firm to the touch and a skewer inserted into the centre of the meatloaf comes out clean. Brush the top with 1 tablespoon of chutney and cook for another 10 minutes—this will give it a nice glaze.

Cool in the pan for 10 minutes. Lift out and place on a cutting board. Peel away the paper and discard.

Cut into six even slices and put two into a container for another meal.

◊ SERVE

Serve 2 slices per person on warmed plates with the rest of the chutney and lettuce tossed in the dressing.

◊ TIPS
- *Two slices of bread will yield a heaped cup of breadcrumbs.*
- *Check the tomato chutney labels for the lowest in sodium for bonus points.*

◊ OPTIONS
- *Garam masala is a blend of about ten spices and could be swapped for a Middle Eastern, Mexican or Indian spice blend.*

SCHNITZEL

This is a great way to enjoy pork on your fork—a great flavour combination.

Pork, potato, carrot and creamy fennel cabbage

Serves 2 • 2230kJ (533 calories) per serve

400g (14oz) lean pork leg steak
¼ green cabbage, about 300g
300g (10½oz) waxy potatoes (about 2), washed
1 large carrot, peeled and sliced
1 tablespoon oil
1 teaspoon fennel seeds
¼ cup light sour cream
1 tablespoon wholegrain mustard or your favourite

◊ OPTIONS
- Red cabbage could be used instead of green cabbage. Canned sauerkraut is good too.
- Sultanas instead of the fennel seeds would go well.

◊ PREP

Trim any visible fat off the pork.

Cut the core out of the cabbage and slice the cabbage into 2cm (¾in) chunks, wash and rinse well. Cut the potatoes into 2cm slices.

◊ COOK

Heat enough water to cover the potatoes in a saucepan with a lid—the water needs to be hot but not boiling. Add the potato and bring the water to the boil. Cover and cook for about 8 minutes, until the potatoes are firm but cooked through.

Add the carrots to the potato for the last 2–3 minutes of the potatoes cooking time. Stick a skewer in the centre of a few pieces of potato and carrot to test if they are cooked.

Meanwhile, heat the oil in a non-stick pan over a medium heat. Add the pork and cook for 3–4 minutes, until golden, then turn and cook for 2–3 minutes; the timing will depend on the thickness of the steaks. Wrap the steaks and pan juices in foil to rest.

Stir the fennel seeds into the pan and as soon as they have released their pungent aroma, stir in the cabbage and cook, stirring, until it is golden—some pieces of the cabbage will be quite wilted and others will still hold their shape. Add the sour cream and about 1–2 tablespoons of water and stir until hot.

Drain the potato and carrot.

◊ SERVE

Place the pork and juices, cabbage, potato and carrot on warmed plates with mustard on the side.

◊ TIP
- *Give the sour cream a good stir before adding.*

MAN SALADS
TOSSED

This makes any piece of meat, chicken or fish more of a meal.

Mixed vegetable salad

Serves 2 • 1212kJ (289 calories) per serve

◊ PREP

Make the salad dressing. Taste and adjust the seasoning as you like.

◊ MIX

Put the lettuce, tomatoes, carrot, onion, red pepper and cucumber in a salad bowl. Toss, using salad servers, to mix well. Add the avocado and mix in the dressing.

◊ SERVE

Serve as a side to grilled, barbecued or roasted meats and seafood.

◊ TIPS
- *Always use the freshest seasonal vegetables available.*
- *Buying pre-washed salad leaves is really time saving (but eat them quickly because they don't last).*
- *If making the salad in advance, cover and refrigerate, then add the avocado and dressing just before serving or else the salad will go soggy.*
- *Instead of slicing the carrot, use a vegetable peeler to cut it into ribbons.*

◊ OPTIONS
- *Use rocket instead of the lettuce. Baby spinach is good too.*
- *Add cooked fresh asparagus instead of the avocado.*
- *Use different coloured peppers—yellow and green and orange—when in season and affordable.*
- *Mix in chopped fresh herbs such as parsley, basil or coriander.*

2 tablespoons Salad dressing (see recipe, page 156)
2 cups mixed lettuce leaves
2 medium tomatoes, quartered
1 carrot, sliced
1 white onion, finely sliced
1 red pepper, sliced
1 cucumber, sliced
½ avocado, chopped

SPUDS

You'd have to search far and wide to find a man who doesn't love his spuds.

Creamy chive, bacon & pinenut potatoes

Serves 2 • 1953kJ (466 calories) per serve

500g (1lb 2oz) potatoes (about 4), unpeeled (see Tips)
3 lean rashers streaky bacon
1 tablespoon mayonnaise
1 tablespoon light sour cream
2 tablespoons pinenuts
2 tablespoons chopped chives

◊ PREP

Cut the potatoes into 1cm (½in) thick round slices. If the potatoes are big, cut the slices in half again so they are mouth-sized. Trim any visible fat off the bacon and chop it into 5mm (¼in) pieces.

Mix the mayonnaise and sour cream together.

◊ COOK

Fill a saucepan with enough water to cover the potatoes and place over heat. When the water is hot but not boiling, add the potatoes and bring to the boil. Put the lid on and cook for about 4 minutes, until the potatoes are firm but cooked through; stick a skewer in the centre of a few to test. Drain and put in a mixing bowl to cool.

Meanwhile, heat a small non-stick frying pan over high heat and add the bacon. Cook, stirring, until the bacon is quite crisp—it will jump around the pan so watch that it doesn't leap right out. Remove the bacon and place in a small bowl.

Lower the heat to low and give the pan a few minutes to cool down. Add the pinenuts and roast, stirring, until they are golden brown—they can turn from golden to black in seconds so watch carefully. Put into the bowl with the bacon.

◊ MIX

Stir the combined mayonnaise and sour cream into the potatoes—use a spatula rather than a spoon so as not to break the slices. Add the bacon, pinenuts and chives, stirring gently to combine.

◊ SERVE

This salad is perfect with cooked or cold meats and seafood. It's a real winner to share at barbecues but you may need to make a double quantity if you have guests.

◊ TIPS
- *Add some canned tuna or salmon in spring water and cherry or grape tomatoes for a light meal.*
- *Buy a good-quality egg mayonnaise rather than a 'light' one—bonus points for finding the brand lowest in sodium.*

◊ OPTIONS
- *Use chopped pecans or hazelnuts instead of pinenuts.*

BEETROOT

There's more to beetroot than burgers with the lot.

Beetroot, spinach, beans and garlic chips

Serves 2 • 806kJ (193 calories) per serve

4 large cloves garlic, peeled
1 tablespoon oil
1 cup canned baby beetroot, drained
400g (14oz) can butter beans, drained and rinsed
1 small red onion, finely sliced
1 cup baby spinach leaves
1 teaspoon red wine or balsamic vinegar

◊ PREP & COOK

Slice each garlic clove into 8 very thin slices.

Heat 2 teaspoons of the oil in a small non-stick frying pan over a medium high heat. Add the garlic to the hot oil, keeping it in a single layer. Cook the garlic until golden brown, turning constantly. Place the cooked garlic on a paper towel to cool; keep the oil to use in the dressing.

◊ MIX

Put the beetroot, beans, onion and spinach in a mixing bowl.

Mix together the cooled garlic oil, the remaining oil and the vinegar. Drizzle it over the salad vegetables and toss using salad servers.

◊ SERVE

Immediately with the garlic chips sprinkled over the top. It goes really well with cooked red meat.

◊ TIPS

- Chewing on fresh parsley helps get rid of garlic breath.
- The salad can be served on its own, in a wrap with Felafel (see recipe, page 140) or with Koftas (page 119) and a dollop of low-fat yoghurt or Tzatziki (page 154).
- For something a bit exotic, toss in peeled sliced oranges and mint leaves.

◊ OPTION

- Use oven-roasted (in foil) baby beetroot when in season. The flavour is quite different, but sensational.

BREAD

A must-have man-salad for your repertoire—quick but impressive.

Olive and garlic bread tomato salad

Serves 2 • 1527kJ (365 calories) per serve

◊ PREP

Preheat the oven to 180°C/350°F/Gas Mark 4. Heat a baking tray on the middle shelf of the oven.

Place the margarine, olives and garlic into a small bowl and mix well. Spread the bread with the olive and garlic spread.

◊ COOK

Put the slices of bread on the heated oven tray and cook 10–12 minutes, until the bread is crisp and golden brown. Remove from the oven and leave on the tray until cold; this will keep the toast nice and crisp. When cold, cut each slice of bread into quarters.

◊ MIX

In a salad bowl, toss together the salad leaves, tomato, cucumber, basil and dressing. Scatter over the olive and garlic bread and feta.

◊ SERVE

This is a great light salad for a meal on its own or it will go with just about any cooked meats.

◊ TIPS

- The end crusts of the bread are great to use for the olive and garlic toast. Wholegrain muffins work well too.
- You could leave out the olive and garlic toast and simply toss the olives through with ripped wholemeal pita pieces.

◊ OPTION

- Vary the salad by using mint instead of parsley and sliced fresh bocconcini instead of the feta. Bocconcini are round balls of soft cheese with a rubbery texture. You can get them at the delicatessen counter or in tubs in the chiller.

1 tablespoon salt-reduced margarine spread

5 small kalamata olives, pitted and finely chopped

2 large cloves garlic, crushed

2 slices wholegrain and oat bread

2 cups torn mixed salad leaves

3 medium very ripe roma tomatoes, roughly chopped

2 medium Lebanese cucumbers, roughly chopped

1 cup torn basil leaves

2 tablespoons salad dressing without herbs (see recipe, page 156)

50g (1¾oz) salt-reduced feta cheese, crumbled

TABOULI

Not just for kebabs!

Mint and parsley cracked wheat

Serves 2 • 943 kJ (225 calories) per serve

½ cup burghul (cracked wheat)

2 teaspoons extra virgin olive oil

1½ tablespoons lemon juice

4 spring onions, trimmed and roughly sliced

2 cups loosely packed parsley leaves, roughly chopped

1 cup loosely packed mint leaves, roughly chopped

2 cloves garlic, finely chopped

4 medium roma tomatoes, quartered

◊ PREP

Pour 1 cup of boiling water over the burghul in a bowl. Stand for about 15 minutes, until it is soft. Drain well.

For the dressing, combine the olive oil and lemon juice in a small bowl.

◊ MIX

Place the burghul, spring onions, parsley, mint, garlic, tomatoes and dressing in a salad bowl and mix well.

◊ SERVE

Serve as a salad, in wraps or as part of a mixed mezze selection.

◊ TIPS

- Chopping the parsley, mint and garlic by hand is great for keeping those muscles toned. If you're in a real hurry, give them a quick whizz in a small food processor. The pros use a mezzaluna.
- If you can grow, beg or steal (with permission of course) freshly picked parsley or mint and tomatoes straight off the vine you will never have tasted such great tabouli.

◊ OPTION

- Use instant couscous instead of burghul.

◊ WHAT IS ...

Burghul (or bourghul) is cracked wheat that has been steamed and dried. It is also known as bulgur (or bulgar).

ONE-POT WONDERS
CHILLI

You can serve this Mexican classic a number of ways.

Beef and bean chilli

Serves 2 • 2529kJ (604 calories) per serve

◊ PREP & COOK

Rinse and drain the kidney beans.

Heat oil in a non-stick medium-sized saucepan over low-to-medium heat. Add onion, capsicum, chilli powder and paprika and cook, stirring, until vegetables are soft. Don't rush it—this may take about 10 minutes and will really develop the flavours.

Add the mince and cook, stirring, for 5 minutes to break up the mince. Stir in the tomatoes and kidney beans and when hot reduce the heat to low, cover and cook for 15 minutes.

Remove from the heat and mix in the parsley.

◊ SERVE

Spoon the chilli into 2 warmed bowls (or a large bowl for scooping and sharing) and serve with torn pieces of pita bread.

◊ TIPS

- DIY chilli powder: blend chilli powder, cumin and sweet paprika to taste.
- Crisp the pita chips by simply toasting the pita bread first—watch it carefully while toasting because it doesn't take long.
- Freeze leftovers in an airtight container—label and date so you know what's in there.

◊ OPTIONS

- If you like to start from scratch (and save a few cents), soak dried kidney beans overnight and cook in lots of boiling water (don't add any salt)—they'll take about an hour. If you make extra, you can freeze them too.
- Serve with steamed rice instead of bread.
- Serve in a soft tortilla wrap with salad.

- 400g (14oz) can kidney beans
- 1 tablespoon oil
- 1 large red onion, finely chopped
- 1 large red pepper, finely chopped
- 2 teaspoons Mexican chilli powder
- 1 teaspoon sweet paprika
- 300g (10½oz) lean beef mince
- 400g (14oz) can diced tomatoes
- ¼ cup chopped flatleaf parsley
- 1 large piece wholemeal pita bread for serving

SHANKS

Feel like a real primal hunter by eating meat with the bone left in.

Lamb shanks and lentils

Serves 2 • 3267kJ (780 calories) per serve

2 x 400g (14oz) frenched lamb shanks
1 cup red lentils
1 tablespoon oil
1 medium brown onion, roughly chopped
1 large carrot, peeled and roughly chopped
400g (14oz) can whole peeled tomatoes, no added salt
½ cup salt-reduced beef stock
2 teaspoons brown sugar
1 tablespoon dried oregano leaves
2 cups baby spinach leaves
2 slices wholegrain bread

◊ PREP

Preheat the oven to 200°C/400°F/Gas Mark 6.

Trim any visible fat from the shanks with a really sharp knife.

Remove any little stones that may have snuck in with the lentils and rinse well.

◊ COOK

Heat a flameproof casserole dish with a tight-fitting lid over a high heat. Add the oil and when it is hot, add the shanks. Brown the shanks all over, turning frequently and watching out for oil splatter. Once the shanks are browned well on all sides, remove the pan from the heat.

Add the onion, carrot, tomatoes, stock, 1 cup water, sugar and oregano to the pan, cover with the lid and place on the middle shelf of the heated oven.

Cook for 45 minutes then take the pan out of the oven and sit it on a wooden board. Turn the shanks with tongs. Stir in the lentils, return to the oven and cook, covered, for a further 45 minutes or until the meat is falling off the bone. Remove from the oven.

Stir through the spinach—there will be enough heat to just wilt it and that's all it needs.

◊ SERVE

Spoon into warmed bowls (you might need two spoons or tongs for the shanks) and serve with the bread at the ready for mopping up all the delicious sauce.

The bones are finger-licking good, so have a bowl of warm water handy as a finger bowl.

◊ TIPS
- *Add extra water when cooked if you would like to have more sauce for mopping up.*
- *Lemon zest and chopped parsley is a great combo to sprinkle over the shanks.*
- *The shanks taste even better if you make them a day before as the flavours develop overnight. They freeze well too.*

◊ OPTION
- *Use parsnip, pumpkin or sweet potato instead of carrot.*

STIR-FRY

The quintessential quick, tasty and healthy meal.

Pork, pepper and ginger stir-fry

Serves 2 • 2224kJ (531 calories) per serve

1 tablespoon brown sugar
1 teaspoon salt-reduced chicken stock powder
2 teaspoons rice wine or malt vinegar
180g (6oz) packet soba noodles
1½ tablespoons oil
400g (14oz) lean pork steak, cut into thin strips
3 small peppers (red, green, yellow or orange), finely sliced
1 large red onion, finely sliced
2 large cloves garlic, finely chopped
3–4cm (1–1½in) piece ginger, very finely sliced

◊ PREP

Get all the ingredients prepped before you even think about firing up the wok.

Make the sauce by mixing the sugar, stock powder and vinegar in a small jug or cup.

Place the noodles in a bowl and cover with boiling water. Stand for 2–3 minutes, then drain thoroughly, gently separating the noodles with your fingers.

◊ COOK

Heat the oil in a large wok over high heat. Test that the oil is ready by dropping in a piece of onion—if it sizzles the oil is ready. Remove the onion.

Add the pork and let the pieces brown before stirring and turning—this will take 2–3 minutes. Stir in the peppers, onion, garlic and ginger and cook, stirring, for 2–3 minutes.

Pour in the sauce and cook for 1–2 minutes until hot, then stir in the noodles. Keep stirring until everything is piping hot.

◊ SERVE

Place in warmed bowls and tuck in with chopsticks—a great way to slow down your eating and enjoy every morsel.

◊ TIP

- If your barbecue has a wok, this is great way to cook for a crowd outdoors.

◊ OPTIONS

- Chicken, beef or fish would be great instead of pork.
- If you use fish, choose a firm-fleshed fish. It's good to cook it first and set it aside in a bowl covered with foil while you stir-fry the vegetables so the fish doesn't break up. Just return it to the wok to heat through at the end.

STEW

The aromatic star anise and the dumplings provide the wonder in this pot.

Slow-cooked beef and coriander dumplings

Serves 2 • 2563kJ (612 calories) per serve

◊ PREP & COOK

Trim any visible fat off the steak and cut into large chunks (about 2cm/¾in).

Heat the oil in a large saucepan with a snug-fitting lid over high heat and brown the meat (see Tip). Reduce the heat to medium. Add the onions to the pan and stir until well browned, about 2 minutes. Stir in the sweet potato, stock, ½ cup water and star anise. Add extra water to cover the meat if needed.

Reduce the temperature to low, put on the lid and simmer slowly for about 1½ hours, until the meat is really tender.

About 30 minutes before the cooking time is up, make the dumplings. Place the flour in a mixing bowl and rub in the margarine with your fingers. Stir in the coriander, egg white and 1–1½ tablespoons water using a round-bladed knife. Mix lightly using clean hands until the mixture forms a ball. Shape into eight even-sized dumplings.

Drop the dumplings into the simmering stew, cover and cook for another 15 minutes—the dumplings will almost double in size as they cook. Turn the dumplings after about 10 minutes cooking time if you like; they'll soak up the stew juices.

Add the beans and steam with the lid on for a couple of minutes, until they turn bright green. Remove the star anise.

◊ SERVE

Spoon the stew and dumplings into warmed bowls and sprinkle with coriander.

◊ TIP
- Don't turn the meat chunks until they move with no resistance. If you tug it, the meat will tear.

400g (14oz) lean blade or topside beef steak
1 tablespoon oil
2 medium brown onions, finely sliced
1 medium gold sweet potato, cut into rough chunks
1½ cups salt-reduced beef stock
5 whole star anise
100g (3½oz) green beans, topped, tailed and halved
2 tablespoons chopped coriander

Dumplings
½ cup wholemeal self-raising flour
2 teaspoons salt-reduced margarine spread
1 tablespoon finely chopped coriander
1 egg white, lightly beaten

CURRY

This curry in a hurry will get you away from the stove and at the table in 30 minutes.

Thai-style chicken curry

Serves 2 (with some leftover, see Tip) • 2518kJ (601 calories) per serve

1 tablespoon oil

300g (10½oz) butternut pumpkin, peeled and cut into 5mm x 1cm (¼–½in) dice

1 brown onion, roughly chopped

1 tablespoon red curry paste

400g (14oz) trimmed chicken breast, cut into 1.5cm (⅔in) cubes

1½ teaspoons brown sugar

1 cup cooked chickpeas, drained (from a can or home cooked)

375ml (13oz) can light coconut-flavoured evaporated milk

250g (9oz) brown 90-second microwave rice

1 cup chopped coriander

1 red chilli, finely sliced (optional)

1 lime, cut into 8 wedges

◊ PREP & COOK

Get everything prepped before you start as this is a very quick recipe to make.

Heat the oil in a non-stick saucepan over a medium heat. Add the pumpkin and cook, stirring occasionally, until golden, about 2–3 minutes, to give it a kick start. Add the onion and stir for 2–3 minutes, until soft.

Stir in the red curry paste and when it is fragrant (about 1 minute), add the chicken and stir for about 3–5 minutes, until cooked.

Add the brown sugar, chickpeas and evaporated milk and bring to the boil. Lower the heat and simmer for 2–3 minutes.

Meanwhile, microwave the rice following the packet directions.

◊ SERVE

Spoon a couple of scoops of rice onto warmed bowls, top with curry and sprinkle over the coriander. Serve with the chilli and lime in a little bowl alongside.

◊ TIPS
- This will make enough curry sauce for three serves so put a third in a container for another day—you could add it to some instant noodles for a quick lunch.
- While you are slowly enjoying the curry, the rice will be absorbing the creamy sauce. Add more chilli or lime juice as you go.

◊ OPTIONS
- Try garnishing with Vietnamese basil, mint or chopped kaffir lime leaves.
- You could use prawns or beef instead of chicken.

CUPBOARD HUNT
SOUP

Make a nourishing snack in an instant.

Egg drop (or egg flower) noodle soup
Serves 1 • 1578kJ (377 calories) per serve

◊ PREP

Make the soup according to the packet directions, then into a small saucepan.

Crack the egg into a bowl and beat lightly

◊ COOK

Bring the soup to the boil over a low heat and cook for about 1–2 minutes. Add the peas and corn, cover the saucepan and cook for about 2 minutes, until the peas have turned bright green.

Pour the beaten egg very slowly into the soup and, at the same time, running the streaming egg through the soup with a fork. The egg will set instantly. Remove the soup from the heat immediately.

◊ SERVE

Pour the soup into a warm bowl and scatter the chives on top. Spread the bread with the margarine and cut into whatever shape you like.

1 packet salt-reduced instant chicken noodle soup-in-a-cup

1 egg

½ cup mixed frozen peas and corn

2 teaspoons snipped chives

2 slices soy and linseed bread

2 teaspoons salt-reduced margarine spread

◊ TIP

If you are making soup for two, double the quantities of all the ingredients except the egg—one egg is still enough for two.

◊ OPTION

For variety, try frozen peas and carrots with parsley, or a small can of chickpeas (rinsed and drained) with some coriander instead of peas and corn with chives.

SPAG-BOL

An all-time favourite with a healthy twist.

Spaghetti and meat sauce

Serves 2 • 2529kJ (604 calories) per serve

1 tablespoon oil
1 medium brown onion, finely chopped
1 large carrot, finely chopped
400g (14oz) lean beef mince
½ cup salt-reduced beef stock
2–3 teaspoons Italian dried herbs
80g (2½oz) wholemeal spaghetti
400g (14oz) can whole tomatoes
20g (²/₃oz) parmesan cheese, finely grated (see Tip)

◊ **WHAT IS ...**
Italian dried herbs are a blend of usually six dried herbs such as marjoram, basil, oregano, rosemary, thyme and parsley. It is sold in supermarkets.

◊ **PREP & COOK**

Fill a medium-sized saucepan about three-quarter full with water and have on standby for the spaghetti.

Heat the oil in a saucepan over a low-to-medium heat (see Tip). Add the onion and carrot and cook for 3 minutes, stirring occasionally. Stir in the mince and cook for 5 minutes, using a wooden spoon to break it up. Stir in the stock and herbs. Cover the saucepan and simmer for 15 minutes.

Meanwhile, bring the water for the spaghetti to the boil (it boils faster if you put the lid on the pot). Add the spaghetti and cook, uncovered, according to packet instructions for timing until al dente.

Stir the tomatoes into the mince and cook, covered, still on low-to-medium heat for 10 minutes.

◊ **SERVE**

Drain the spaghetti into a colander and divide between warmed serving bowls. Spoon over the sauce and sprinkle with parmesan.

◊ **TIP**

- Packaged finely grated parmesan cheese is available; however, you may prefer to purchase a slice off the block and grate it finely yourself—20g equals 4 teaspoons.

◊ **OPTION**

- Use fresh oregano, parsley and basil instead of dried herbs but add them right at the end of cooking time to preserve their colour.

Belly-busting Recipes

RISOTTO

This Italian staple will give you real Master Chef cred.

Smoked paprika marinara risotto

Serves 2 • 2566kJ (613 calories) per serve

◊ PREP

Dissolve the stock in 1 cup boiling water.

Dry the seafood on a paper towel and keep in the fridge until required.

◊ COOK

Heat 1 tablespoon of the oil in a large saucepan over a low-to-medium heat. Add the onion and rice and cook, stirring, for 2 minutes. Stir in the stock, tomatoes and the paprika and bring to the boil. Put the lid on the saucepan and turn the heat down to low. Cook for 20 minutes, giving the rice a stir every 5 minutes. Stir in the peas for the last 5 minutes of cooking time.

Meanwhile, heat the remaining oil in a heavy-based non-stick pan over a medium-high heat. Put the larger pieces of seafood into the pan first and after a few minutes add the smaller pieces. Make sure the seafood is spread out well for even cooking. Cook until golden on each side—try to turn each piece only once.

Stir the seafood and the dill gently through the rice.

◊ SERVE

Place the rice into warmed bowls with lemon wedges on the side.

- 1 teaspoon salt-reduced chicken stock powder
- 400g (14oz) seafood marinara mix (see Tip)
- 1½ tablespoons oil
- 1 large red onion, finely sliced
- ½ cup arborio rice (see Option)
- 100g (3½oz) canned diced tomatoes
- 2 teaspoons smoked paprika
- 1 cup frozen peas
- 1–2 tablespoons finely chopped dill
- 1 small lemon, quartered, pith and seeds removed

◊ TIPS
- You can buy seafood marinara mix at the supermarket or fishmonger.
- You can make this easy risotto just with prawns or your favourite seafood. Sliced chicken breast fillets works well too.

◊ OPTION
- You can use parsley, coriander or chives instead of dill.
- You could replace the lemon with a lime.

◊ WHAT IS ...

Traditionally, arborio rice is used to make risotto. It makes a creamy dish. You could also use short-grain (calrose) or low-GI rice. Arborio is medium GI.

FELAFEL

One of the great foods of the Mediterranean ...

Sesame chickpea balls

Makes 20 balls; 10 balls to serve 2 & 10 balls for later on   •   1982kJ (473 calories) per serve

¼ cup sesame seeds
400g (14oz) can chickpeas, rinsed and drained
1½ cups frozen peas
2 large cloves garlic, peeled
2 tablespoons self-raising flour
2 teaspoons baharat spice blend (see Note)
1 tablespoon oil
2 small wholemeal pocket breads
1 cup Tabouli (see recipe, page 154)
3 tablespoons hummus (see recipe, page 151)
3 tablespoons low-fat natural yoghurt

◊ PREP

Dry-roast the sesame seeds in a small heavy-based non-stick frying pan over a medium heat for 3–5 minutes, until golden brown. Stir while cooking and keep a watch so they don't burn. Tip them into a bowl.

Whizz the chickpeas, peas, garlic, flour and baharat in a food processor, blending until well mixed for about 1 minute.

Shape the mixture into 20 balls a little smaller that the size of golf balls. Dip the balls into the sesame seeds and roll them around until well coated.

◊ COOK

Wipe out the frying pan with a dry paper towel. Heat half the oil—test that it is hot enough by dropping in a few leftover sesame seeds; if they sizzle the oil is ready. Remove the sesame seeds otherwise they'll burn.

Place half the balls in the pan and cook until golden brown all over. You'll need to turn them often. Set aside the cooked balls to cool them on a plate covered with a paper towel. Heat the remaining oil and cook the rest of the balls.

◊ SERVE

Arrange the balls on plates with the pocket bread, tabouli, hummus and yoghurt.

◊ TIPS

- Baharat (a Lebanese spice blend) gives Middle Eastern dishes a distinctive aroma and flavour. The spice is available from good spice shops, online or you can make your own using the recipe on page 153. Keep some in the cupboard.
- The cooked felafels freeze well.

◊ OPTIONS
- *It's OK to use ready-made tabouli to save time*
- *Served with Tzatziki (see recipe, page 154) as a dip, these make great party platter finger food.*

PIZZA

Once you've made your own, it's hard to go back to the mass-produced stuff.

Crisp-base sardine, tomato and rocket pizza

Serves 1 • 3132kJ (748 calories) per serve

100g (3½oz) piece wholemeal pita bread
1 tablespoon salt-reduced margarine spread
1 tablespoon no-added-salt tomato paste
200g (7oz) tomatoes, finely sliced
100g (3½oz) can sardines in spring water, drained
40g (1½oz) salt-reduced feta cheese, crumbled
1 cup baby rocket leaves
1 small lemon, quartered, pith and seeds removed

◊ PREP

Preheat the oven to 180°C/350°F/Gas Mark 4, then heat a baking tray on the middle shelf of the oven.

Spread the bread with the margarine.

◊ COOK

Place the bread on the heated baking tray and cook for 5 minutes, then remove the tray from the oven.

Spread the tomato paste over the base—a spatula works well—and arrange the tomatoes on the top in a single layer.

Bake in the oven for about 8 minutes, until the tomatoes are hot and the base crisp. Transfer the pizza to a large, clean wooden board. Arrange the sardines over the tomatoes (they don't need cooking) and scatter the feta and rocket on top.

◊ SERVE

Serve on the board and cut into wedges with a sharp knife. Garnish with lemon wedges—the juice squeezed over the pizza is delicious.

◊ TIPS

- *This is a great way to use up any over-ripe tomatoes—use roma (egg-shaped), cherry (round baby ones), grape (tiny egg-shaped) or a mixture of them all.*

SWEETS
SUNDAE
Life is sweeter with mulled cherries on top.

Mulled cherries and almond
Serves 2 • 866 kJ (207 calories) per serve

◇ PREP & COOK

Remove the stones from the cherries if you like. Use an olive stoner—it's a handy gadget—or cut through the centre of the cherries to remove the stones.

Put the cherries, 1 cup of water, the sugar, cinnamon stick and cloves in a small saucepan over medium heat. Stir until the sugar has dissolved—this will only take a minute or so. When the mixture comes to the boil, reduce the heat to low and put a lid on the saucepan. Cook for 5 minutes then take off the lid and increase the heat to high.

Stir constantly until the sauce reduces by about half and is syrupy. If you're not sure if the sauce has reduced enough, test it by placing a small amount on a cold saucer—if you can run your finger through the centre leaving a clean line, the syrup is ready.

Take the cherries off the heat immediately and cool.

◇ SERVE

Discard the cinnamon stick and cloves and divide the cherries between two tall glasses or sundae dishes. Top with the yoghurt. Drizzle over the syrup and sprinkle the almonds on top.

150g (5oz) cherries (see Option)
1 cup water
1½ tablespoons brown sugar
1 cinnamon stick
10 whole cloves
4 scoops low-fat frozen vanilla yoghurt
2 tablespoons toasted flaked almonds

◇ TIPS
- *The cherries and syrup will thicken on standing. If this happens, just add a little boiling water and stir.*
- *You could serve the cherries warm with low-fat yoghurt or custard.*

◇ OPTION
- *Use canned cherries in juice when cherries are out of season.*

FRUIT

This recipe is a simple way to enjoy the goodness of seasonal fruit.

Amaretti peaches and yoghurt

Serves 2 • 1220kJ (291 calories) per serve

2 large yellow or white peaches
1 cup low-fat vanilla yoghurt
½ cup Amaretti crunch (see recipe, page 145)

◊ PREP

Cut the peaches into halves and remove the stones. Peel if desired.

◊ SERVE

Place the peaches in dessert bowls. Spoon over the yoghurt and sprinkle with Amaretti crunch.

◊ TIP

- *Peaches are more flavoursome at room temperature but on a hot day they are great served chilled.*

◊ OPTIONS

- *Replace peaches with any fresh seasonal stone fruit such as nectarines or apricots, canned fruits in natural juice (pears are good), or thawed frozen fruits such as raspberries, blueberries or mixed berries.*
- *Serve with low-fat ice cream or custard instead of yoghurt for a change.*

CRUNCH

You'll want to add this delicious and versatile topping to everything once you taste it.

Amaretti crunch

Makes 1½ cups /6 x ¼ cup serves • 567kJ (135 calories) per serve

◊ PREP

Preheat the oven to 180°C/350°F/Gas Mark 4.

Place the amaretti biscuits in a small plastic bag. Crush into small pieces with a rolling pin.

Line a 27 x 17cm (11 x 7in) rectangular baking pan with baking paper.

◊ MIX

Place the flour and margarine in a bowl. Mix, using a pressing action with the back of a wooden spoon, until the mixture is combined and looks lumpy. Stir in the crushed amaretti biscuits, oats and sugar.

Tip the mixture into the prepared baking pan and tap pan on the bench to spread it out evenly.

◊ COOK

Place the baking pan on the middle shelf of the oven. Cook for 10 minutes before stirring the mixture well and cooking for about another 5–10 minutes, until golden brown. Cool.

◊ SERVE

Sprinkle the crunch over any fresh or stewed fruits, ice cream or yoghurt.

◊ TIP
- Store the Amaretti crunch in an airtight container in the kitchen cupboard for up to a week.

◊ OPTION
- Use low-GI sugar, brown sugar or coffee sugar instead of raw sugar.

50g (1¾oz/18 small) amaretti biscuits
⅓ cup plain flour
2 tablespoons margarine spread
2 tablespoons traditional rolled oats
1½ tablespoons raw sugar

◊ WHAT IS ...

Amaretti are small Italian biscuits made with almonds, sugar and egg whites. They are crunchy and lower in fat than regular biscuits.

CRUMBLE

A great comfort pud for a chilly night. No fighting. There's a pot for each person.

Rhubarb crumble with walnuts
Serves 2 • 1449kJ (346 calories) per serve

1 cup Stewed rhubarb (see recipe, page 147)
¼ cup self-raising flour
1 teaspoon cinnamon
¼ cup chopped walnuts
1 tablespoon brown sugar
1 tablespoon margarine spread
2 scoops low-fat vanilla ice cream

◊ PREP

Preheat the oven to 210°C/410°F/Gas Mark 6.

Spoon the rhubarb evenly into two ovenproof 1-cup dishes.

Place the flour, cinnamon, walnuts, sugar and margarine in a bowl. Mix, using a pressing action with the back of a wooden spoon, until the mixture is well combined and looks lumpy.

Sprinkle the crumble evenly over the top of the rhubarb.

Place the dishes on a baking tray.

◊ COOK

Bake for 15 minutes, but keep checking to make sure the crumble topping isn't browning too quickly (cover it with foil if it is) and the rhubarb is not bubbling over.

Remove and let stand for a few minutes before serving or else they will burn the roof of your mouth.

◊ SERVE

Top with a scoop of ice cream or serve the ice cream in a small dish on the side.

◊ TIP
- Make this crumble when your oven is already on roasting meat or whatever—it saves energy.

◊ OPTIONS
- Use finely sliced raw, cooked or canned apple instead of rhubarb.
- Use any stewed fruits in season—stewed quinces make a really great crumble.

RED FRUIT

Stewed rhubarb

Makes 6 x ½ cup serves • 183kJ (44 calories) per serve

◊ PREP & COOK

Trim the leaves from rhubarb and chop off any damaged ends. Cut the rhubarb into 4cm lengths.

Put the rhubarb, sugar and ½ cup of water in a saucepan. Cook over a low-to-medium heat until it starts to simmer. Reduce the heat to low and simmer for 10–15 minutes, stirring occasionally.

◊ SERVE

Eat the rhubarb on its own, with low-fat ice cream, yoghurt or custard, or use as a base for a crumble, top muesli or porridge with it or whatever takes your tastebuds' fancy.

1 bunch rhubarb
3 tablespoons sugar

PUDDING

You'll be bowled over by this little pud's rich chocolatey taste.

Self-saucing chocolate pudding with orange
Serves 4 • 1007kJ (241 calories) per serve

1½ tablespoons margarine spread
¼ cup sugar, plus 1 tablespoon
½ teaspoon vanilla extract
1 egg, lightly beaten
½ cup self-raising flour
3 teaspoons cocoa powder
1 tablespoon reduced-fat milk
2 medium oranges
4 small scoops low-fat vanilla ice cream

◊ PREP

Preheat the oven to 180°C/350°F/Gas Mark 4.

Rub four 150ml (¼pt) ovenproof dishes with margarine.

Cream the margarine, ¼ cup sugar and vanilla in a small bowl using a handheld mixer—it will only take a minute or two—then beat in the egg.

Sift together the flour and 2 teaspoons of cocoa and add to the egg mixture with the milk (use a cake scraper). Mix until smooth.

Divide the mixture among the greased dishes.

Combine 1 tablespoon of sugar and the remaining cocoa and sprinkle the mixture evenly over the puddings. Give the dishes a gentle tap on the bench to spread out the sugar mixture evenly.

Pour an equal amount of boiling water carefully and evenly into each dish (about 1½ tablespoons in each)—it's a good idea to pour the water over the back of a spoon to break the impact of the water hitting the top of the mixture.

◊ COOK

Place the puddings on the middle shelf of the oven and cook for 15–20 minutes. Test if they are ready by inserting a cake tester in the centre—if it comes out clean the puddings are cooked; alternatively, just touch the top of the puddings and if they're firm and the sauce is bubbling they're done.

Stand the puddings for about 10 minutes before serving.

◊ SERVE

Meanwhile, peel, quarter and remove any seeds or pith from the oranges. Cut the flesh into bite-sized pieces.

Place each pudding dish on a plate with the orange and ice cream on the side.

◊ TIPS

- *Cocoa powders vary a lot in flavour and the price is not always a guarantee of richness and flavour. Try a few until you find one that's really satisfying—bitter, sweet and chocolaty.*
- *Naval oranges are great for this recipe—they're easily peeled, seedless and very juicy.*

ICE

This will make a good impression at your next summer soiree or romantic dinner.

Mango and apple granita

Serves 2 • 756kJ (181 calories) per serve

1 cup chilled apple and mango fruit juice or other combined juice mixture

1 tablespoon sugar

1 medium mango, peeled and cut into small cubes

few sprigs of fresh mint, very finely chopped

2 scoops low-fat vanilla ice cream

◊ PREP

To make the granita, put the juice and sugar in a small saucepan. Stir over a low heat until the sugar dissolves.

Pour the juice into a 20cm (8in) round pan and cover with plastic wrap. Put the pan into the freezer and set a timer for 1 hour. Check to see if ice has started to form. Once it has, scrape the ice with a fork. If it is sloppy rather than icy, just give it a stir. Cover again and return to the freezer.

Set the timer again for 1 hour and again scrape the ice with a fork. Repeat this process each hour another three or four times. Each time you give it a scrape, the ice particles get smaller and the mixture has a creamier look and texture. It is a long process but is well worth the effort.

Transfer the granita to a suitable container and store in the freezer until required.

◊ SERVE

Pile the mango into two glass bowls or cocktail glasses. Sprinkle with the mint and top with the ice cream.

◊ TIP

- *The granita can be served on its own or with different fruit and a scoop of low-fat ice cream as a hot-weather snack.*
- *Another great combo is cranberry fruit juice granita with chilled watermelon.*

◊ OPTION

- *If you have an ice cream machine, freeze the granita following the manufacturer's instructions.*

FANTASTIC FLAVOURS
HUMMUS

This Mediterranean dip is more than a dip—it makes a great spread for rolls and sandwiches and can even be served as a 'sauce' with meat or chicken dishes.

Chickpea and garlic dip

Makes about 1½ cups

◊ PREP

Rinse and drain the chickpeas.

◊ MIX

Place the chickpeas, garlic, oil, tahini paste, cumin and lemon juice in the bowl of a food processor or blender. Process until well combined, about 1–2 minutes.

Add 1–2 teaspoons of water and process until quite smooth. Add extra water if needed to get the texture right.

◊ SERVE

Serve with torn pita bread as a dip and part of a mixed (mezze) plate or spread on wraps and sandwiches.

◊ STORE

Keep the hummus in a covered container in the fridge for up to a week and use as required.

400g (14oz) can chickpeas (see Tip)
3 cloves garlic, peeled
2 tablespoons extra virgin olive oil
1 tablespoon tahini paste
½ teaspoon ground cumin
1 tablespoon lemon juice

◊ TIP

- *You can prepare your own dry chickpeas by soaking overnight and boiling in plenty of fresh water for around an hour, until tender. They can then be frozen in small quantities without liquid in sealed freezer bags—it's a good idea to flatten the bag for quick freezing, thawing and for freezer stacking. Label and date them ready for adding to soups, salads or curries.*

◊ WHAT IS ...

Tahini is a paste made of sesame seeds. There are two choices—hulled or unhulled. Unhulled is more nutritious. Once opened, keep tahini in the fridge.

DUKKAH

This nutty/seedy Middle Eastern mix adds zing and crunch to almost anything but traditionally is served with bread and oil for dipping

Hazelnut and spice mix
Makes 1 cup

¼ cup hazelnuts
¼ cup sesame seeds
1½ tablespoons cumin seeds
2 tablespoons coriander seeds

◊ TIPS
- Keep a small coffee grinder specifically for grinding spices. Or clean out your coffee grinder with bread before using it for spices—and clean it again carefully after using so your coffee is not tainted with the spice flavours.

◊ OPTION
- Substitute pistachio or pine nuts for the hazelnuts.

◊ PREP & COOK

Dry-roast the hazelnuts in a heavy-based non-stick pan over a medium heat for about 10 minutes, stirring occasionally so they brown evenly. Keep an eye on them so that they don't burn. Remove the nuts and place on a paper towel. When they are cool enough to handle, rub to remove the skins.

Reduce the heat to low and add the sesame seeds to the pan. Toast until golden, 5–10 minutes, stirring often. Place in a small dish.

Add the cumin seeds to the pan. Toast for about 2 minutes, stirring, until they release a toasty aroma. Place in a separate dish.

Add the coriander seeds to the pan. Toast for about 2 minutes, stirring. The aroma will alert you to when they are done. Place in another dish.

◊ MIX

Place the hazelnuts in the bowl of a small food processor and process until roughly chopped. Add the cumin and coriander seeds and process for about 15 seconds. Add the sesame seeds and process for another 15 seconds.

◊ STORE

Place into a covered container and store in the fridge.

◊ USES

Sprinkle over salads, mix into meat dishes and add to dressings—a great substitute for salt.

BAHARAT

Ian (Herbie) Hemphill is an absolute legend in the spice trade, and he's happy to share the love of spices.

Herbie's Lebanese seven-spice mix

Makes 2 heaped tablespoons

◊ MAKE

Blend the spices together carefully.

◊ STORE

Keep the spice in a clean small glass jar in the cupboard.

◊ TIP

- Baharat is the perfect spice blend to rub on lamb before roasting or grilling or to add to slow-cooked lamb dishes.

Recipe courtesy of Ian Hemphill, Herbie's Spices at www.herbies.com.au.

4 teaspoons mild paprika
2 teaspoons ground black pepper
1 teaspoon ground cumin
1 teaspoon ground coriander seeds
1 teaspoon ground cassia
½ teaspoon ground cloves
½ teaspoon ground cardamom seed

TZATZIKI

Sure you can buy it, but this is easy, cheaper and tastes so much better.

Yoghurt and cucumber dip

Makes 1¼ cups

¼ cup finely chopped or grated cucumber, skin on and seeds removed

1 cup low-fat plain yoghurt

1 clove garlic, crushed

◊ PREP

Squeeze any excess liquid from the cucumber using kitchen paper towel.

◊ MAKE

Mix the yoghurt, cucumber and garlic in a bowl until well combined.

Store in a covered container in the fridge for up to a week.

◊ USES

Dollop on hot and cold cooked meats and fish, as a dip for prawns, vegetable sticks and torn pita bread or as a spread on sandwiches and wraps.

◊ TIPS

- *Add some finely grated lemon or lime zest—it's particularly good with seafood.*
- *Freshly shredded mint or basil can be stirred through just before serving.*

◊ OPTIONS

- *You can leave the seeds in the cucumber if you like and are going to make and serve the tzatziki straight away.*
- *You can increase or decrease the amount of garlic to suit your taste.*

AIOLI

Aioli is the best thing since ... well, sliced bread.

Garlic mayonnaise

Serves 2

◊ MIX

Put the garlic, lemon juice and mayonnaise into a small food processor or blender. Blend until well mixed—it will take less than a minute.

◊ SERVE

Dollop it on or use as a dip for cooked prawns, serve on jacket potatoes or use on Steak and prawns (see recipe, page 116).

2 large cloves garlic, peeled
1 teaspoon lemon juice
1½ tablespoons mayonnaise

◊ TIPS

- *Aioli is best freshly made and eaten.*
- *If you're not a gadget person, mix the Aioli by hand in a small glass bowl with a whisk.*
- *Buy good-quality mayonnaise—look for the one that's the lowest in sodium.*

◊ OPTION

- *Finely shredded mint or basil can be mixed into the Aioli.*

SALAD DRESSING

I've never met a vegetable that doesn't taste better without dressing—use this and eat more vegetables.

Olive oil, vinegar and herb dressing

Serves 2

1½ tablespoons extra virgin olive oil

2 teaspoons balsamic or red wine vinegar

½ teaspoon Dijon or wholegrain mustard

freshly chopped or dried herbs—parsley, mint, basil or dill, optional

¼–½ teaspoon sugar, optional

few grinds of black peppercorns

◊ MAKE

Put the oil, vinegar, mustard and herbs in a plastic lidded screw-top jar.

Shake to combine. Add the sugar and pepper and shake again. Taste the dressing and adjust seasonings as you like.

◊ SERVE

Toss it through salads and drizzle it on salad ingredients or cooked vegetables.

◊ TIPS

- You can transform this dressing into many others by changing the ingredients—try raspberry, white wine or malt vinegar and hazelnut or walnut oil, or a combination of extra virgin olive oil with a dash of chilli oil.
- Mix dressings in a small bowl or cup—a small whisk is ideal.

GRAVY

Pass the gravy ... and not the one out of a box.

Nutty brown gravy

Makes 2/3 cup

◊ COOK

Place the oil and flour into a small saucepan over a medium heat and, stirring vigorously and constantly, cook for 3–5 minutes, until the mixture turns dark brown. Remove from the heat.

1 tablespoon oil
1 tablespoon plain wholemeal flour

Add 1 cup of water very gradually, stirring all the time. The mixture will thicken and then go very thin again—it must be stirred constantly. Return the saucepan to the heat and stir until it comes to the boil. Continue stirring and boiling until reduced by about one third.

Strain the gravy through a fine sieve into a bowl if you would like smooth gravy but the husks of the flour can be left in for some fibre. Reheat if needed.

◊ SERVE

Hot over roasted meat and vegetables.

◊ TIP
- *Patience is needed to make this gravy if you want it to be lump-free.*

◊ OPTIONS
- *Mustard gravy—add smooth or grainy mustard to taste.*
- *Redcurrant gravy—add redcurrant jelly to taste.*
- *Herb gravy—toss in some very finely chopped parsley or chives.*

SAUCE

Mint sauce always reminds me of Sunday lunch with the family

Traditional mint sauce—sweet and tart

Makes 4 serves

2 tablespoons white sugar

2 tablespoons chopped mint

2 tablespoons malt vinegar

◊ MAKE

Dissolve the sugar in 1 tablespoon of boiling water in a heatproof jug. Add the mint and vinegar and leave to cool.

◊ SERVE

Stir well before serving with roast lamb.

◊ TIP

- *Taste the sauce and adjust flavours if needed.*

PART 5

HOW TO LOVE FOOD
& BUST YOUR BELLY

In this section I give you the belly-busting basics:

- The best foods for a bloke's body—foods you need to eat every day
- Putting it on the plate—eating the right foods in the right ratio
- Steer-clear foods—learning the numbers that really matter
- The biology of belly busting—how to outsmart your primitive brain
- Handling hunger—tips for taming the hunger beast
- The brain and belly busting—how to get your head around it.

You get out of your body what you put in. Food is fuel power. Bodies, like cars, need the right mix of fuel for best performance and regular maintenance to stay running smoothly.

THE BEST FOODS FOR A MAN'S BODY

Get the group benefits with:

- meaty foods
- bread and grains
- fruit and vegetables
- dairy foods
- the good oils
- water

Power up the machine with protein

What? Red meat, pork, chicken, fish, seafood, eggs and legumes (beans, lentils and chickpeas).

Why? Protein gives you muscle power. It helps to build and maintain strength (and make running repairs). It's also good for shutting up the hunger rumbles.

How? Keep it lean and medium sized.

Re-fuel the machine with carbs

What? Grain foods such as bread, rice, pasta, noodles, couscous and breakfast cereals; and starchy vegetables like spuds and sweet potato.

Why? Your body revs on carbs. They are the energy foods your brain and body need to run. The slow burning, high fibre ones (usually brown or wholegrain) will also help bust your belly because they fill you up, give you staying power (and keep you regular).

How? Medium-sized portions are enough.

FORGET LOW-CARB

It's a fad. It's pretty hard to stick to for any length of time and comes with some rather unpleasant side effects like a fuzzy brain, bad breath and constipation. Instead, go for slow-burn low-GI carbs when you can. I tell you about them on page 176.

And forget about ... the 'no carbs after 5pm' rule. Just cut back a bit and avoid the nocturnal square-eyed pig-out on junk. (Find out more on pages 54 and 62.)

Rust-proof the body with fruit and veg

What? Vegetables such as carrots, tomatoes, onions, broccoli, mushroom, lettuce, celery, courgettes, pumpkin, parsnips, peas, peppers, corn, broccoli, cabbage, beans and beetroot. Fruit and berries such as apples, oranges, bananas, pears, grapes, kiwifruit, plums, nectarines, rockmelon, papaya (paw paw), mango and strawberries.

Why? The vitamins, minerals, fibre and phytochemicals (fight-o-chemicals) they contain stop you falling apart from the inside and make you feel great. They are your belly-busting best friends—offering so much for so little cost (in kilojoules/calories).

How? Pile your plate high with veggies (but be moderate with dressings and sauces) and crunch a couple of pieces of fruit a day.

Reinforce the frame with good dairy foods

What? Milk, yoghurt, cheese and custard.

Why? Dairy is the best source of calcium to your keep bones and teeth strong but also choc-full of essential vitamins and minerals to toughen your man-frame. They're great for belly busting because they satisfy hunger, provide longer lasting energy and better blood sugar (glucose) levels.

How? Enjoy three serves a day and make 'em low fat. For example, one cup of light milk, one tub of light yoghurt and one slice of light cheese is three serves.

Does milk give you a belly-ache?

You may not have enough milk-digesting enzyme but don't worry—you can drink soy milk instead, and make sure it has calcium added. Dairy yoghurt and cheese should be OK.

FUNNY THAT ...
Market research says men buy more carrots than any other vegetable because they're simple to prepare and can be served raw or cooked. These little babies are idiot-proof—you can even serve them half-cooked. Men also like their food spicier than women.

WHAT ABOUT ...
Butter and cream (and sour cream) are bad dairy foods. They are fats, and the artery-clogging kind. So is coconut cream and coconut milk.

COLOUR CODE

The colour of your meal is a good indication of how healthy it is. Contrasting colours are good. Monotone is not. For example a pie and chips are the same colour, nutrient deficient and fattening (but OK once in a while).

CHOOSE BETTER

If you're out and about or on the road and need food fast and your only option is the food hall, corner shop or takeaway, steer clear of the monotone deep-fried nasties. Have the hamburger instead (one pattie is plenty) with egg and salad but skip the bacon, cheese and fries.

On page 68 we have listed some great eating out options.

Grease the machine with the right oils

What? Oils such as sunflower, olive and canola; spreads like margarine or peanut butter; nuts and seeds, and avocado.

Why? Good oils are liquid-gold goodness and provide essential fats and vitamins, lower cholesterol and add great flavour and enjoyment to meals.

How? Don't go overboard—you don't need a lot.

Grease line

If you've ever let a fast-food box of deep-fried chicken go cold, you'll notice a solid white grease slick at the bottom of the box. This is also what fast food does to your arteries. The same with other foods high in saturated fats such as the fat on meat, butter, cheese (but you can eat lower fat ones; see above), cream, cakes and pastries.

US research has found men who eat the most saturated fats have poorer semen quality, whereas those who ate more polyunsaturated fats—in fish, grains, seeds and nuts—had the best quality sperm. Foods such as fried chicken, chips, pies and burgers not only make you slow and sluggish but knock out and slow down your swimmers as well.

Prevent overheating with fluids

What? Water, juice, cordial, tea and weak coffee.

Why? A man can't be at his best in drought conditions. For best performance drink at least 2 litres (5 pints) of fluids a day—more in hot weather and during exercise. How? Make it mostly water and choose low-sugar options to bust that belly.

PUTTING IT ON THE PLATE
Make a meal of it
To bust your belly you need to eat foods from each group every day in the right ratio.

WRONG RATIO
a plate full of spaghetti with meat sauce

RIGHT RATIO
half a plate of spaghetti bolognaise with half a plate of salad
or a small bowl/plate of spag bol and a bowl of salad

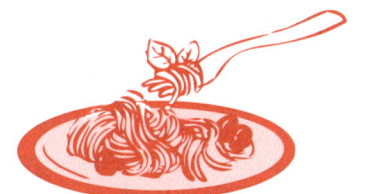

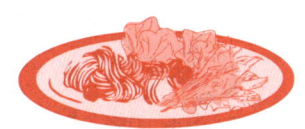

Eat foods in the right ratio
1. Make a **quarter** of your meal power protein: meat, chicken or fish.
2. Make another **quarter** carb fuel: pasta, bread, noodles or potato
3. Aim to fill **half** your plate with vegetables (and not all the same one), raw or cooked.

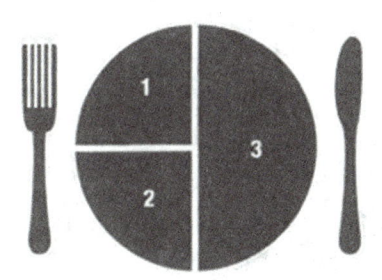

You can do this at home, when you buy food out and about, and when you're ordering at restaurants. If you're still hungry, eat more vegetables.

How to Love Food & Bust Your Belly

Rough it

Your insides will work better and you'll bust your belly sooner if you eat lots of foods with roughage (dietary fibre).

What? Breakfast cereals with bran and wholegrains, wholemeal and mixed grain bread, legumes (beans, lentils and chickpeas), vegetables, fruit and nuts.

Why? Eating foods with fibre is like taking a mop and broom to your intestines and giving them a good clean out. You'll pass number twos more often and with ease. You'll feel lighter and brighter. Foods with fibre also help fill you up so it's easier to eat less.

Eating more fibre is easy as changing your cereal or bread.

STEER-CLEAR FOODS

It's good to focus on the positive—all the great foods you can and should eat every day when you are belly busting. But it's probably handy to be reminded of the keep-it-for-a-treat-foods. That means:

- cakes, biscuits, slices, muffins, doughnuts
- chocolate and/or cream biscuits
- chocolate and chocolate bars
- cream, sour cream and butter
- fast food, chips and pies (anything deep fried)
- potato and corn chips (anything salty in a packet)
- alcohol
- soft drinks, flavoured mineral water, sports drink and ice tea (diet or light is OK).

GOOD OPTIONS FOR SHARE PLATES

Sharing plates (multiple small portions rather than individual meals)

Asian: Rice paper rolls, Thai beef salad; steamed rice, stir-fries.

Greek (mezze): Greek salad, bread & dips, vine leaves, grilled prawns or octopus, grilled meats and vegetables (souvlakia), beans (fassiola).

Lebanese (meze): tabouli, bread and dips, kibbeh, stuffed cabbage leaves, broadbeans, meat skewers (shish kebab), grilled chicken (shish tawook).

Spanish (tapas): Green salad, olives, meatballs, mushrooms, roasted peppers (pimento), tortilla (potato omelette), paella.

BURN OFF

Fattening foods go down so fast—but, boy, they have staying power if you want to burn them off. This table gives you an idea how long you would have to walk at an average walking speed (4 kilometres per hour) to burn them off.

If you eat...	the burn-off time walking will take	because the energy intake in kilojoules to work off is	you are eating the following % of total DI all in one go
1 slice chocolate mud cake (200g/7oz)	174 minutes	3630	42%
1 jam doughnut	58 minutes	1210	14%
caramel nougat chocolate bar (53g/1¾oz)	50 minutes	1050	12%
4 chocolate-coated cream biscuits	72 minutes	1499	17%
1 piece fish plus chips	122 minutes	2533	29%
fried chicken and chips	146 minutes	3044	35%
big burger meal (big burger, large chips and cola)	235 minutes (almost 4 hours!)	4897	56%
100g bag potato chips	102 minutes	2130	24%
750ml (24fl oz) bottle cola	60 minutes	1260	14%

What does this table mean?

Bad food choices quickly add up to centimetres around your belly and take a lot of exercise to get rid of—it's easier not to do the damage in the first place rather than try and fix it afterwards.

DON'T BE FOOLED ... IT'S ALL CAKE

A cake by any other name has just as many kilojoules.

- A muffin is just a cake baked in a muffin tray.
- Banana bread is not bread. It's just a cake baked to look like a loaf.
- Date loaf is a cake baked in a loaf tin.
- Carrot cake is not a serving of vegetables. It's cake.

Men can strip down engines, build bridges, fly aircraft, market products, manage projects, budgets and people. You need to apply some of this nous to organising your food and exercise—it's not brain surgery.

✸ Re-engineering tips

Most men just eat whatever is in front of them. If you're eating fattening, less healthy foods every day, it's time to re-engineer your life to ensure they're not in front of you and something better is.

- Don't keep these foods in the house, office or desk.
- Don't let yourself get hungry enough to grab just anything.
- Shop regularly so you have healthy food on hand.
- Don't buy your usual or what your mate's getting, look for healthier options.
- Pack your own lunch for work.
- Avoid situations where fattening foods are hard to avoid.

Slouch potato

Eaten in front of the telly, food you eat goes straight to your belly. Eating while watching TV is a double whammy: you will eat mindlessly (probably on unhealthy fattening food you see advertised) plus your metabolic fuel burn slows right down to a level not much higher than sleeping. To bust your belly, avoid eating in front of the TV.

A moment of taste, a lifetime of waist.

BOOZE-BUSTING

Many men love their beer, others prefer spirits or wine. Whatever your tipple, you need to cut back on booze to bust your belly. Alcohol is a rich fuel source and you need to work hard to burn it off.

Going cold turkey is perhaps an unrealistic choice, but it will make the biggest dent in your belly (especially if you eat better food as well). If you're doing the Top gear belly-busting programme (see page 13), you need to avoid alcohol during this phase. However, if you're happy with a steadier approach, then just cut back on what you're having now.

You don't need to ban the booze—just cut back.

In case you didn't know, men are recommended to limit alcohol to three to four units a day and have two alcohol-free days a week.

One unit equals 10ml or 8g of pure alcohol—for example:

- 1 x single (25ml) measure of whiskey (ABV 40%)
- $1/3$ pint of beer (ABV 5–6%)
- 1/2 standard (175ml) glass red wine (ABV 12%)

Three to four units is equal to a pint and a half of 4% beer.

Check the volume of alcohol in your drink. Some beers may have 3.5% alcohol, but stronger ones may contain 5 or 6 % ABV. The alcohol content of wines may be as high as 17% ABV.

NUMBER CRUNCH

The unit of alcohol is based on the volume of alcohol a drink contains—this is called Alcohol By Volume (ABV).

✹ Drink tip

The number of units of alcohol it contains is listed on the container of an alcoholic beverage.

How to Love Food & Bust Your Belly

How much is that drink worth?

Going over the top with booze is not only a massive calorie blow-out with zero nutritional return, but you're more likely to choose bad food and not feel like exercising the next day.

A 375ml (12fl oz) bottle or can of beer contains 570kJ—about the same as two slices of bread. If you drink one a day surplus to your energy (kilojoule) needs, this is enough to gain 6kg (13lb) and around 4cm (1½in) around your waist in a year.

Booze and belly busting

- If you drink every day, cut back to four days a week (and so on).
- If you usually drink four, drink two.
- Buy your beer in smaller amounts (it will stay colder when consumed slowly).
- Pour your beer and wine into smaller glasses at home.
- Try light beers until you find one you like.
- Find a soft drink you can order at a bar (eg, soda, lemon, lime & bitters, diet cola—not juice because it has just as many kilojoules as beer).
- Drink water or soda water between glasses of wine.

Men's wisdom—what works

Phil, aged 40, company director
A vigorous exercise regime and smaller portions works every time. There are no silver bullets—just commit to the process and you will be successful.

Don, aged 72, retired businessman
Give priority to eating food that is minimally processed—or as close to its original form as possible. Eat heaps of fruit and vegetables.

GET REAL

So many men have an all-or-nothing approach to eating and exercise: you're either a fully charged, starving gym-junkie teetotaller, or you're eating and drinking with a devil-may-care twinkle in your eye.

An all-or-nothing approach does not work. You need to embrace the idea that any improvement is progress. Don't be so darned perfectionist—it's not helping.

Richard, aged 35, teacher
Low-GI cereal or oats for breakfast. Keep carbohydrate portions modest at dinner (and stick to low-GI ones). Almost never have puddings, chocolate, cake, sweets or chips. Do some exercise almost every day.

Alan, aged 64, retired public servant
Keep exercising, and most of the time keep some restraint on diet. Be vigilant about using low-fat and low-GI foods.

Old-fashioned belly-busting wisdom—still pure gold

- Eat breakfast.
- Eat your vegetables.
- It's not dinner time—get out of the kitchen!
- You can't eat all that.
- Serve yourself a smaller amount and go back for seconds if you're still hungry.

No, no, no ... forget it

- Finish everything on your plate.
- Chubby is healthy.
- Accept everything you're offered to be polite.
- If you love me, you'll eat it all.
- You can start your diet tomorrow.
- ... I'm a growing boy (yeah, outwards).

THE BIOLOGY OF BELLY-BUSTING

NUMBER CRUNCH

Every kilogram (2lb 3oz) of fat on your body stores around 32,500 kilojoules (7760 calories). That's the equivalent of 87 cans of beer, 31 chocolate bars or 30 packets of chips. To lose the fat, eat less treats.

Belly busting is much like balancing the books—you need to know how much is going in (food) and how much is going out (exercise). To shrink your belly you need to go into the red. To maintain a smaller belly you need to hover around the break-even point.

Belly basics

There's no mystery about going up trouser sizes over the years. From a physiological point of view, food is fuel and your body is a very efficient machine that has stored excess fuel when you didn't need it. A big belly means you've been eating more than you need for a while.

In order for the stored fat around your waist to be used for fuel, you need to create a fuel shortfall; eat fewer calories, and burn more calories by moving more.

Men's wisdom

Phil, aged 40, company director

You are like a car and food is fuel. Everything you eat needs to be burnt off. Fill the tank with food and you need to drive around to burn it off. If you leave the car parked in the garage, the tank stays full.

Food vs exercise

Unless you have the time and energy to do a *Biggest Loser*-style boot-camp programme, you need to eat less. The majority of your belly-busting progress will be from eating better food and taking care to eat the right amounts. There is no getting around the fact you will feel hungry—at least for a while. The human body is programmed to protect its current weight, even if this is an XL-sized belly. You need to outsmart your primitive biology.

Doing some exercise and generally being more active will accelerate your progress. Exercise also helps maintain muscle, which burns fuel at a higher rate even when you're sitting still. This means when you've got muscle on board you can eat more without gaining weight. This will help maintain your belly-busting progress. Being active also makes you feel good, and puts you in a better mood.

Men's wisdom

Tristan, aged 25, legal research clerk
Eating well and exercise need to be done together to be effective. If you eat healthier foods that you aren't that keen on and don't exercise, it's harder to see results and the better food is harder to take. And vice versa: if you work out and hate it, but still eat the foods that are adding to your waist, then the exercise is being wasted. If you do both, you'll be happier with your results and the sacrifices you make will seem all the more worth it.

Eat just enough to get you through to your next meal.

Filling up the tank

Food is your fuel and to keep your belly busted in the long term you need to learn how to refuel according to the distance you travel. Unlike off-road vehicles with additional fuel tanks you fill to go farther between stops, the human body does best on a drip-feed system and regular stops.

If you overfill your tank, all else being equal, you'll simply store it away. If you do overfill your tank from time to time, eat less at the next meal and/or do more exercise to use up the extra.

Men's wisdom

Charles, aged 52, carpenter
I used to have a big dinner and never felt like eating breakfast when I got up the next day. I used to work until 9.30am and then pig-out on coffee and doughnuts or shocking stuff like cookies and chocolate bars. I tried a smaller dinner and—surprise, surprise—I felt hungry in the morning and had a good breakfast that saw me through to lunch. That one change made a big difference for me.

DON'T BE FOOLED
A hard belly is not better than a soft one—in fact, quite the opposite. A hard belly means every one of your fat cells is swollen to its maximum size and the skin is stretched to fit them in. A soft belly means the fat cells have started to shrink. You cannot lose fat cells (unless you suck 'em out with cosmetic surgery), but you can make them much smaller and look better in your clothes.

NUMBER CRUNCH

Both these foods have the same number of kilojoules but vastly different nutrient content.

1050kJ (251 calories) caramel nougat chocolate bar

- protein 2g (1/10oz)
- fat 9.5g (1/3oz)
- insignificant levels of vitamins and minerals

1143kJ (273 calories) light chocolate milk

- protein 15g (½oz)
- fat 8g (¼oz)
- vitamins A, B12, riboflavin
- calcium, phosphorous, potassium, magnesium, zinc

The milk is by far the most nutrient-dense option. The other difference between these two foods is their different filling power. A chocolate bar doesn't fill you up as well as chocolate milk does.

Choose quality fuel

If you want the best performance from your body, you need to choose good-quality fuel. Put simply, 'you are what you eat'—what you swallow today, shows up tomorrow. A long career of swallowing bad foods has added up to your reflection in the mirror today, but what has been done can be undone.

In fuel for motor vehicles, octane level is important; in fuel for men, nutrient density is key.

Nutrient-dense foods offer more 'bang for your calorie buck'— they burn better and more cleanly.

What is... a nutrient?

Nutrients are the components of food the body uses to stay healthy. Nutrients include water, protein, carbohydrate, fats, vitamins and minerals.

Nutrient-dense foods are 'core' foods (the ones we said you need to eat every day, see pages 58–61), whereas nutrient-poor foods are often called junk foods.

Choosing nutrient-dense foods puts some nutrition backing behind the calorie numbers.

You're better off chugging low-fat flavoured milk (see Number Crunch, left) than chowing-down on the chocolate bar. Although they have the same kilojoule content, the milk is more nutrient dense and more filling so you can successfully eat less over the day.

A matter of taste

Many men choose junk food because they say it tastes better; however, this is an example of the need to outsmart primitive human biology. The urge to consume fatty, sweet and salty foods was of benefit to our hunter-gatherer ancestors but is now a distinct disadvantage. You need to re-train your sense of taste. Taste buds adapt in around four weeks to appreciate the taste of real food rather than the hyper-intense flavours of junk food.

WHAT IS ...

GI stands for Glycemic Index and relates to carbohydrate foods. The GI of a food is the degree to which it increases your blood glucose levels during digestion. High-GI foods are digested and absorbed quickly, spiking blood glucose levels and the (fat-storage) hormone insulin. Low-GI foods are better because they release their energy more slowly and it lasts for longer. Eating lower GI foods also helps maintain steady blood sugar, insulin and energy levels.

HANDLING HUNGER

Optimal fuel for the human male is the kind that burns slowly and lasts longer. Quick-burning fuel will go up in smoke, leaving you grabbing a nutrition disaster at the nearest corner store or vending machine.

Slow-burn fuels are low-GI foods and protein foods.

Low-GI foods

The best way to lower the GI of your diet is to choose lower GI options of everyday foods, such as bread, breakfast cereal and potatoes — they satisfy your hunger to help bust your belly.

Legumes (beans, lentils, chickpeas), milk products, oats, pasta and most fruits have a low GI. When it comes to grain foods, lower GI options are generally — but not always — those that have been less processed. The GI does not apply to meat because that has almost zero carbohydrate.

HIGHER GI FOOD	LOWER GI ALTERNATIVE
puffed rice cereal, corn flakes	rolled oats (porridge), muesli
jasmine rice	basmati or low GI-rice
white bread	multigrain, dense grainy breads
Maris piper, Desiree potatoes	Nicole, Marfona, Estima, new potatoes (all boiled)
mashed potato	butternut pumpkin, carrot or parsnip

Source: GI rankings from www.glycemicindex.com

The power of protein

One of the biggest snags during belly busting is feeling hungry. But this can be minimised by ensuring there is protein in your fuel mix. Protein-rich foods seem to keep your stomach busy and quiet for longer. But there's no need to go berserk and drink protein powders and eat only chicken breasts and egg whites. Balance and variety are still important principles to follow.

How to: protein power your meals

Breakfast: include milk, yoghurt, eggs, legumes or nuts, eg:
- porridge or muesli with milk or yoghurt
- poached egg or baked beans on wholegrain toast
- skim-milk fruit smoothie
- fruit salad with low-fat yoghurt sprinkled with nuts and seeds.

Lunch: include lean meat, fish, egg, chicken or legumes, eg:
- roast beef and salad roll
- sardines on toast
- grilled chicken and vegetable sandwich.

Dinner: include lean meat, chicken, fish, egg or legumes, eg:
- grilled steak, potato and vegetables
- barbecued fish fillet with bread roll and salad
- stir-fry pork, noodles and vegetables
- lentil burger with salad.

Snacks: include milk, yoghurt, legumes or nuts, eg:
- low-fat yoghurt
- low-fat milk (plain or flavoured)
- unsalted almonds or peanuts
- hummus dip with wholegrain crackers.

You can harness the belly-busting power of protein by including protein from healthy sources at every meal.

✷ Tips for fighting off the hunger beast

- Re-programme yourself to believe hunger is not bad, but a sign of progress (each hunger pang is a fat cell shrinking).
- Have a tall glass of water before you eat.
- Eat more slowly to give your brain a chance to register you've had enough. Focus on eating. Concentrate on enjoying each mouthful and chewing it well.
- Once you've finished your meal, pack all the food away and vacate the kitchen. Get into doing something else to distract yourself from eating food you don't need, such as reading, puzzles, cards, DIY, working on the car.
- After your meal, chew sugar-free gum or brush your teeth to signal eating time is over.
- Make a rule: you do not eat in front of the TV.

THE BRAIN AND BELLY BUSTING

If I had a dollar for every time I heard a man say 'I know what I should be doing, I just don't do it' you'd be getting this book for free!

The way I see it, there are two reasons this happens: either you can't or you won't. I hope I can help with the 'can't' by teaching you how to choose better food in every situation, but overcoming the 'won't' is a bit trickier—just giving you more knowledge doesn't work. You have to change your mind.

Life is not a race to the finish, and neither is a healthy life. Think of it as a nice drive to be enjoyed—some parts of the journey will be more scenic and exciting than others, but it all adds up to a great trip.

Busting your belly will take a fair bit of blood, sweat and tears. It helps if you can see the overhauled 'waistline winner' version of yourself in your mind so you can do the work. This is the belly-busting man's equivalent of the carrot and the donkey ...

Men's wisdom
Kim, aged 40, defence force aircrew
Get off your arse, don't be scared to exercise, talk to people who can help. Start slowly with exercise—you don't have to be an iron man to be a man. Don't beat yourself up if you slip backwards. Just take some pride in yourself.

BELLY-BUSTING GUIDE TO PUTTING YOUR MIND IN GEAR

1. **Commit**
   - Decide that you want to bust your belly and be healthier.
   - Remind yourself often of the benefits.
   - If you falter, get back on track.

2. **Get real**
   - Forget about *Biggest Loser*-style results—such dramatic change is impossible under normal circumstances.
   - Decide what changes are realistic and possible for you and consolidate these over time.
   - Cut down slowly on fattening food or drink you love or swap it with something healthier.

3. **Focus on the positive**
   - Accept you are imperfect and so are your eating habits and lifestyle.
   - Believe that small changes add up over time.
   - Focus on what you can eat, not on what you can't/shouldn't.

4. **Be accountable**
   - Tell those close to you of your intention to bust your belly and be healthier (they'll probably help or even join you).
   - Keep track of your waist over time (once a month).
   - Take a series of 'after' photos to document progress.

✱ Electronic tip

Smart phones are great for keeping track of your waist measurement and your food, drink and exercise. In psychology-speak this is called self-monitoring and it works a treat to keep you honest and on-track.

Are you stuck?

If you're stuck in old habits and sick of others 'nagging' about change, it may be time to take a long, hard look at what is really important in your life. Is it your family, your career, or just having a good time? It is sobering to think about how your life would change if your health took a turn for the worst. Men tend not to value their health until it goes wrong. But without health there can be no work and no play—just existence with imitations. Nobody thinks ill-health will happen to them. Newsflash: no-one is bullet-proof. Don't leave change until it's too late.

Where are you now?

In order to make changes, you need to know the state of play right now. A good way to do this is to keep a food and exercise diary: a bit like a logbook for your car (see over the page). You can buy food and activity diaries in newsagents and bookshops, and phone apps are available too, but you can also make your own. The following is a format you can use. There is a blank version you can photocopy on the next page.

How did you get here?

It might help, but it is not essential, to explore how your trousers got to be so large and why your belly has expanded over the years. It's not essential because some men just want to get on with it. Others will benefit from thinking more about the causes to help fix them. Did your belly expand because you stopped exercising? Is it because your job now requires you to eat out with clients or travel a lot? Have you been hitting the booze? Have you been using food for emotional comfort or reward? Having you given up on cooking and surviving on take-away?

All these causes have slightly different solutions but overall you have to care for yourself and see yourself as worth the effort.

MEN'S WISDOM

Michael, aged 38, retail manager

'I've turned over a new leaf and can't believe I waited so long to change my terrible lifestyle. I feel so much better eating healthy food and walking every day. I've lost 5cm (2in) from my waist and would like to lose another 5. I want to see my kids grow up and be able to play with them and coach them at footy. My wife suggested I take a "before" photo and I refused at the time but now I wish I had so I had a record of how far I've come.'

FOOD & EXERCISE DIARY

Time	Food type and amount	Comments	Exercise type and duration
7.30am	1 bowl of cornflakes and milk 1 glass of orange juice	in a hurry	walk 10 minutes to train station
11am	cup of tea 2 plain sweet biscuits	hungry, and biscuits provided at work	
1pm	takeaway stir-fry noodles and chicken orange juice	chicken had skin and not many vegetables—no time to make my lunch this morning	
4pm	packet of potato crisps can of soft drink	peckish, from vending machine	walk 10 minutes from station
7.30pm	cheese and crackers lasagna (frozen) garlic bread (frozen) peas and corn (frozen) glass of red wine	v. hungry, couldn't wait for dinner wine helps me relax	
9.30pm	handful of milk chocolate-coated licorice	watching TV and relaxing	

FOOD & EXERCISE DIARY

Time	Food type and amount	Comments	Exercise type and duration

Change the record

Everyone has voices in their head and these are actually your thoughts to yourself. Have you ever stopped to listen to your thoughts? Are they helpful or critical? If the main voice in your head is an a***hole, then this might be affecting how you act, including what you eat and how you look after yourself generally. It is possible to change the thoughts in your head by just being aware of them and thinking differently. You men might say you can handle a bit of nasty, but we all know you catch more flies with honey than vinegar (and you're all big softies inside).

Men's wisdom

Walter, aged 58, nurse

'My problem was food was my old and trusted friend that stuck with me through crappy times at work, a relationship breakdown and the death of both my parents. I could always rely on it as a cheap and reliable 'hit' of happiness, even when everything else was turning to s***. But over the years I just got bigger and bigger and my back started to pack it in. With the help of a psychologist and a dietitian provided through work, I realised food is no way to deal with emotional stuff, and it left me in a worse state. I had to learn to look for other means of emotional support. I've learned to communicate a lot better with those close to me and my weight has gradually come down, although I still have a way to go. I now feel ready for a new relationship.'

✸ Tip

Remember, you don't have to take on all these changes at once, but choose a few things at a time and build on these.

How to use your food and exercise diary to change

Identify problems

- Are your portions too large?
- Are you eating too much junk food?
- Are you eating too many fatty fast foods and takeaway foods?
- Are you drinking too much alcohol?
- Are you spending too much time sitting?

Identify opportunities

- Are you eating enough wholegrain foods and vegetables?
- Are you drinking enough water?
- Are you eating enough fruit and fish?
- Are you eating any legumes or nuts?
- Are you getting enough exercise?

PART 6

WAIST MATTERS

For those of you who are interested, in this section we explain the health effects of a big belly.

- Why bellies expand.
- Why is a big belly so bad?
- When is a belly too big?
- What the hell is BMI and why should you care?
- Big bellies and survival of the species.
- Bellies and bad blood.
- Why are you still hungry?

In medical terms, a big belly is known as 'central obesity'. Fat stored around the middle increases your risk of high cholesterol, heart attack, diabetes, high blood pressure and bowel cancer.

NUMBER CRUNCH

Surveys suggest that two-thirds of men (67%) are fatter than is good for them, and men are fatter than women (52%). Getting older compounds the problem—a slim man over 55 is hard to find.

WHY BELLIES EXPAND

It happens to the best of men: footy stars, cricketers, politicians, businessmen teachers and tradies. No particular group is spared. You might laugh it off with 'it's all muscle' or 'it's genetic', but when people ask when the baby's due it's not that funny. Unfortunately, men tend to store fat around their middle—where it wreaks the most health havoc.

So why are so many of you expanding around the middle? Why is there so much more of you to hug these days?

It's not just one thing, its lots of things all happening together that make it harder to stay in the same size trousers. The sheer numbers of men with big bellies suggest there are powerful forces at play. The way we live has changed.

- Jobs are no longer physical and we prefer to sit down and relax in our spare time. For many men, there is no necessity to move much at all.
- Fattening food is everywhere and it's often easier to eat it than not.

You could just give up and say 'that's life', but we all know that being large comes at a high cost. The fact is you feel better, look better and live longer if you're smaller around the middle.

The world is kinder to men who aren't fat too: they have better jobs, earn more money and attract more women.

WHY IS A BIG BELLY SO BAD?

Besides looking unflattering, a big belly is a health risk. As well as filling those fat cells under the skin until they're ready to burst, this so-called 'visceral' fat also nestles itself around your organs.

Even if you sucked out your belly fat with liposuction, you'd still have the troublesome fat around your organs. The only way to get rid of that is to burn it off with the right diet and exercise.

As well as being more comfortable in your clothes, busting your belly will make you feel younger, more energetic and more ready to meet the challenges life throws at you. It will also improve your love life (more on this later).

NUMBER CRUNCH
According to a recent Australian study, 27% of adult males are classified as too big around the middle, increasing their risk of disease.

In general, a healthy waistline is less than 94cm (37in) for men (80cm/31½in for women). The bigger your waist, the bigger your risk.

Measure your waist
1. Grab a tape measure, preferably a soft one (ask the lady of the house).
2. Stand naked and wrap the tape around your middle (or, better still, have your partner do this for you).
3. Align the tape with your belly button and ensure it is the same level all the way round.
4. Take a deep breath in, and let it out again. Pull the tape until it is snug but not tight.
5. Read the measurement.

If you don't have a soft tape measure but have a hard metal builders' tape, use a piece of string to do your waist and then measure it along the builders' tape to get your measure.

WHAT IS BMI?
You've probably heard of the Body Mass Index (BMI), which is your weight in kilograms divided by your height in metres (squared). For example (105kg = 230lb):

105kg ÷ (1.72 x 1.72) = 35 BMI

BMI 18.5–24.9 = ideal
BMI 25–29.9 = overweight
BMI 30 or more = obese

There are shortcomings to the BMI for assessing fatness. For example, if you're highly muscled (a weight lifter or front-row forward), your BMI will not distinguish between higher muscle weight and fat.

The BMI is used for collating national statistics. It is not perfect, but it does give a pretty good estimate of the number of people carrying much more weight than is good for them.

NUMBER CRUNCH
Three-quarters of men over 55 are overweight (BMI 25+) and one in three men over 55 is obese (BMI 30+).

> **The waist measure, however, eliminates the margin for error in the BMI and is a very good measure of fatness.**

BMI and ethnicity

There are different waist targets for some ethnic groups. If you have a South Asian (eg, Indian), Chinese, South-east Asian, Central or South American background, your waist target is lower at 90cm (35½in) rather than 94cm (37in). This is because you tend to store fat around your belly (you are more apple shaped) at a lower weight.

> **Having skinny arms and legs does not make a pot belly any less harmful.**

Because there are such large numbers of failed dieters, it's obvious there's more than lack of will-power going on. There are powerful forces throwing a spanner in the works of good intentions. Belly busting is your guide to neutralising these forces to allow your healthy body to triumph. We'll teach you how to outsmart a fattening world.

Men's wisdom
Scott, aged 43, carpenter
I am worried about my waist at my age as it could be a bit smaller and my mum has diabetes. I have lost weight before by drinking less beer and not eating so much fatty food. What has stopped me is my love of beer and my social life! My advice? Do what's best for you: sometimes just cutting back and doing some sit-ups is all it takes.

Big bellies and survival of the species
If you were paying attention in biology class at school, you'd know about Darwin's theory of evolution and 'survival of the fittest'. But in the case of humans, in the past it may well have been 'survival of the fattest'.

Until the introduction of modern agriculture around ten thousand years ago, humans were hunter-gatherers. They had to deal with periods of feast and famine, and in these conditions fatness was an advantage to see you through hungry times. The human body may be in fact be hard-wired to keep you fat in case of famine.

Of course, if you're lucky enough to live in an affluent country, famine is history and we live in a permanent state of feasting. Unfortunately, we're not cut out for this and thus a permanent state of fatness wreaks havoc with our health. In this day and age, fatness is a distinct disadvantage—chances are you'll be afflicted with chronic disease and die younger.

Big bellies and bad blood
You might think your belly just sits there minding its own business, but you'd be wrong. The fat stored there is actually making trouble all the time. You can't feel it, but your fat has a secret life making hormones to muck up your metabolism.

DON'T WAIT TILL IT'S BROKE
Guys are famous for not going to the doctor until things are grim. Please regard your body as you would a motor vehicle: although regular servicing requires investment, it reduces the risk of bigger, more expensive problems later ... and it ensures a smooth ride and optimal performance. Doctors aren't that bad. Get to know yours and visit once a year, even if all is well. Fill out your logbook with vital stats such as blood pressure, cholesterol, blood glucose and waist measure.

In medical lingo, it's called **metabolically active tissue**. This is how it's possible for a big belly to be so bad for you. Your big belly and the problems it causes may mean you have the metabolic syndrome (Syndrome X). The metabolic syndrome puts you at high risk for developing a heart attack or type 2 diabetes.

Have you got it?

You qualify as having the metabolic syndrome when your waist is greater than 90cm (35½in) plus any two of the following:

- high blood triglyceride level (>1.7mmol/L)
- low (good) HDL cholesterol level (<1mmol/L)
- high blood pressure (or you are taking medication for this)
- raised fasting blood glucose level (>5.6mmol/L, or you already have type 2 diabetes).

These numbers are obtained with a blood test and blood pressure measurement. If you don't know your numbers, make an appointment with your doctor to fill in the gaps. Don't have a doctor? Get one.

If you have the metabolic syndrome, consider it a direct message from your maker that you are neglecting or mistreating your equipment and you're warranty is now void. You can fix it, yes you can. You need a food and movement overhaul—and there's no time like the present.

Bellies and blood sugar

Blood sugar is actually glucose that comes from the food you eat. Glucose is the body's primary fuel source and is transported around the body in your blood. Normally it is kept within a tight range by a hormone called insulin but a big belly stops insulin

> If famine ever happens, it is some consolation that the big-bellied men will survive. In the meantime, you need to crack the metabolic code and do some re-wiring to bust your gut. It can be done through modifying what you eat and working your body in the right way.

working properly. This is called 'insulin resistance' and leads to blood glucose levels becoming too high. After a while, this can turn into full blown type 2 diabetes—and that usually ends up needing medication, or ultimately insulin injections.

The great news is, the runaway train to diabetes can be pulled up by busting your belly fat, feeding yourself right, and moving your body more. And, if you already have diabetes, busting your belly can make your diabetes disappear.

Bellies and blood fats

Why a big belly causes your blood fats to go up is really quite obvious. A big belly means your body is awash with spare fuel (food) and it's using your belly as a storage depot—like a camel stores water in its hump. Some of this spare fat can spill over into your blood. A high triglyceride level basically means there's an oil slick in your pipes. When the pathology lab spins down your blood for testing, a layer of fat settles on the top like the cream from a bottle of milk straight from the cow. A high cholesterol level happens in much the same way.

A big belly doubles your chances of high cholesterol.

Bellies and blood pressure

When you are large, you have more blood to supply the extra bulk. Your heart then has to work harder to get the blood around. It pumps with greater pressure. On top of this, your blood vessels become less elastic—meaning they cop the full force of each beat rather than rolling with the punches. This contributes to heart attack, stroke and kidney damage.

Men's wisdom

Aaron, aged 42, IT executive
I'm worried about my waist because any increase in my waist size seems inversely proportional to my ability to pull

hot chicks. I've tried reducing my waist in the past but have achieved mediocre results. What helped me was envisioning hot chicks fancying me, but sometimes the effort was too much. I'd rather not give any advice to other men about busting their belly because it just creates more competition!

Why are you still hungry?

In a remarkable twist of fate, having a big belly does not mean you are less hungry.

In fact a big belly may make you hungrier when any fool could see you've had more than enough to eat.

Part of the reason for this paradox is your brain doesn't seem to get the same 'I'm full' signals when your belly fat is stopping your insulin from working properly (this is called 'insulin resistance'). On the flip side, you can reduce insulin resistance by busting belly fat, eating the right foods and moving more.

> Having a big belly and being physically inactive increases the risk of erectile dysfunction. Busting your belly and exercising help you keep 'up'

Blokes' wisdom

Kim, aged 40, defence force aircrew
I equate a larger waist with being unfit and it ties strongly to my self-worth, and my professionalism. In aviation we are required to be fit, and there is peer pressure to maintain fitness.

FURTHER INFORMATION

Don't just wing it with your health

KNOW YOUR NUMBERS
They tell you things about your health you need to know.

Waist size (men)
Increased risk: more than 94cm (37in)

Greatly increased risk: more than 102cm (40in)

Heart health
- Blood pressure
    - Less than 140/80 (over 65 years)
    - Less than 130/85 (under 65 years)
- Triglycerides < 2.0 mmol/L
- Total cholesterol < 4.0 mmol/L (<5.5 if no other risk factors*)
- HDL (good) cholesterol > 1.0 mmol/L
- LDL cholesterol < 2.5 mmol/L (may be <3.0 if no risk factors)

*Risk factors are overweight/obesity, high blood pressure, type 2 diabetes, smoking, history of heart disease (heart attack/angina), high alcohol consumption, insufficient physical activity, kidney disease

Diabetes
- Fasting blood glucose

Diabetes ≥6.1 (or ≥10.1 two hours after glucose drink test)

Pre-diabetes

Impaired Glucose Tolerance ≤ 6.1 (and ≥ 6.7 and <10 two hours after glucose test)

Impaired Fasting Glucose ≥ 5.6 and <6.1 (between 6.1 and 6.7 two hours after glucose test)

Cancer

- PSA (ng/ml)

    Less than 2 (age 40–49)

    Less than 3 (age 50–59)

    Less than 4 (age 60–69)

    Less than 5.5 (age 70–79)

Numbers you need each day

- 2 & 5 serves of fruit and vegetables
- 8 hours sleep
- At least 30 minutes physical activity/7000–10,000 steps

CHECK IT OUT

Each year you need

Age 20–39

- Check up with your GP
- Skin exam
- Dental exam and cleaning
- Self-examination of testicles for lumps

Age 40–49

- Check up with your GP
- Skin exam
- Dental exam and cleaning
- Self-examination of testicles for lumps

Age 50–64

- Check up with your GP
- Skin exam
- Dental exam and cleaning
- Eye test
- PSA test
- Self-examination of testicles for lumps

65 and over

- Check up with your GP
- Skin exam

- Dental exam and cleaning
- Eye test
- Hearing test
- Flu shot
- PSA test
- Self-examination of testicles for lumps

Tests/shots to discuss with your GP for the 50s and over

- ECG
- Cholesterol
- Diabetes (fasting blood glucose)
- Bone density
- Bowel cancer screening
- Immunisation review
- Pneumonia shot

FIND OUT MORE

There's lots of great information around to help you keep yourself in good condition.

Find a dietitian

- British Dietetic Association <www.bda.uk.com> and click on 'Find
- American Dietetic Association <www.eatright.org>
- Dietitians of Canada <www.dietitians.ca>

Exercise specialists & information

- Chartered Society of Physiotherapy <www.csp.org.uk> and click on 'find a physio'
- Get a life, get active <www.getalifegetactive.com>
- The Register of Exercise Professionals (REPS) <www.exerciseregister.org>
- Physical Activity Guidelines for Americans <www.health.gov/paguidelines>
- American Society of Exercise Physiologists <www.asep.org>
- American Physical Therapy Association (APTA) <www.apta.org>
- Canadian Physiotherapy Association <http://thesehands.ca>
- Canadian Society for Exercise Physiology <www.csep.ca/english>
- The Certified Professional Trainers Network <www.cptn.com> and click on 'find certified trainers'

Men's health

- Men's Health UK <http://menshealthuk.net>
- Health of men <www.healthofmen.com>
- Centers for Disease Control (CDC), Men's Health <www.cdc.gov/men>
- National Institutes of Health, Men's health <http://health.nih.gov/category/MensHealth>
- Health Canada, Just for you-men <www.hc-sc.gc.ca/hl-vs/jfy-spv/men-hommes-eng.php>
- Men's Health Canada <www.menshealthcanada.com>

Heart health

- British Heart Foundation <www.bhf.org.uk>
- American Heart Association <www.heart.org/HEARTORG>
- Heart and Stroke Foundation <www.heartandstroke.com>

Diabetes

- Diabetes UK <www.diabetes.org.uk>
- American Diabetes Association <www.diabetes.org>
- Canadian Diabetes Association <www.diabetes.ca>

Mental Health

- Mental Health Foundation <www.mentalhealth.org.uk>
- Mind-For better mental health <www.mind.org.uk>
- National Institute of Mental Health <www.nimh.nih.gov>
- Canadian Mental Health Association <www.cmha.ca>

Cancer

- Cancer UK (directory) <www.cancer-uk.org>
- American Cancer Society <www.cancer.org>
- Canadian Cancer Society <www.cancer.ca>

Food & nutrition guidelines

- British Nutrition Foundation <www.nutrition.org.uk>
- Food Standards Agency <www.food.gov.uk>
- Nutrition information and guidelines <www.nutrition.gov>
- Health Canada- Food and nutrition <www.hc-sc.gc.ca/fn-an/index-eng.php>

Glycemic Index

- Glycemic Index Database **<www.glycemicindex.com>**
- Glycemic Index Symbol Program **<www.gisymbol.com>**
- Glycemic Index Laboratories (Toronto) **<www.gilabs.com>**

Quitline

If you need help to stop smoking call

- UK **0800 022 4 332;** USA **1877 448 7848**; Canada **1866 318 1116**

ACKNOWLEDGEMENTS

Thanks to all the men in our lives who have provided so much inspiration and so many insights for this book. We are also grateful to the men who gave permission for their stories to be used in the hope of helping others.

We are forever grateful to Philippa Sandall for her brilliant guidance, ideas, suggestions and general positivity. Thanks to the staff at New Holland: Mary Trewby for her light-touch editing that kept our straight shooting 'bloke-talk' style and the support and encouragement from Diane Jardine. We'd also like to thank Fiona Schultz for her ongoing faith in our books.

Thank you to Diane Temple for her quick and easy meal suggestions, to exercise physiologist Miriam Chin for her exercise information and to Ian 'Herbie' Hemphill from Herbie's Spices for his excellent herb and spice blends.

INDEX OF RECIPES

Aioli 155

Amaretti crunch 145

Amaretti peaches and yoghurt 144

Bacon 'n' egg brekkie 91

Baharat 153

Beans 97

Beef and bean chilli 131

Beef and lentil meatloaf 122

Beef 107

Beetroot 128

Beetroot, spinach, beans and garlic chips 128

Bix, fruit and pecans 89

Bread 129

Burgers 117

Capsicum 1121

Cereal 89

Chickpea and garlic dip 151

Chicken 108

Chilli 131

Couscous 110

Creamy chive, bacon & pinenut potatoes 126

Crisp-base sardine, tomato and rocket pizza 142

Crumble 146

Crunch 145

Cumin potatoes, carrot and bean couscous 110

Curry 136

Cutlets 120

DIY baked beans 97

Dukkah 152

Egg drop (or egg flower) noodle soup 137

Egg, dukkah mayonnaise and rocket wrap 99

Eggs 93

Felafel 140

Fish 'n' chips 106

Fruit 144

Fry 91

Garlic mayonnaise 155

Gravy 157

Hazelnut and spice mix 152

Herbie's Lebanese seven-spice mix 153

Honey mustard glazed pork kebabs 118

Hummus 151

Ice 150

Kebabs 118

Koftas 119

Lamb and pesto penne 101

Lamb cutlets and eggplant dip 120

Lamb in pita with tabouli and yoghurt 119

Lamb shanks and lentils 132

Lamb 104

Mango and apple granita 150

Meatloaf 122

Melt 92

Mint and parsley cracked wheat tabouli 130

Mix 88

Mixed vegetable salad 125

Mulled cherries and almond 143

Mushrooms 95

Mustard and horseradish beef salad 98

Noodles 100

Nutty brown gravy 157

Oats with honey and rhubarb 90

Olive and garlic bread tomato salad 129

Olive oil, vinegar and herb dressing 156

Open beef burger with egg 117

Pasta 101

Pizza 142

Pork, capsicum and ginger stir-fry 134

Pork, potato, carrot and creamy fennel cabbage 124

Porridge 90

Potatoes 113

Pudding 148

Raisin, cranberry and walnut grain-ola 88

Red fruit 146

Rhubarb crumble with walnuts 146

Rice 102

Risotto 139

Roasted capsicum with onions and garlic 112

Roll 98

Salad dressing 156

Salmon with lemon dill yoghurt 96

Salmon 96

Salmon, chips and salad 106

Sauce 158

Schnitzel 124

Scrambled eggs with spinach, walnuts and feta 93

Self-saucing chocolate pudding with orange 148

Sesame chickpea balls 140

Shanks 132

Sherry and smoked paprika mushrooms 95

Slow-cooked beef and coriander dumplings 135

Smoked paprika marinara risotto 139

Soup 137

Spag-bol 138

Spaghetti and meat sauce 138

Spiced Moroccan chicken with lemon 108

Spuds 126

Steak 114

Steak, prawns and aioli 116

Stew 135

Stewed rhubarb 146

Stir-fry 134

Studded rosemary and garlic leg of lamb 104

Succulent roast beef 107

Sumac slow-roasted tomatoes with avocado 94

Sundae 143

Tabouli 130

Tandoori chicken rice 102

Thai-style chicken curry 136

The perfect barbecue steak 114

Tomato, basil, bean and two cheeses 92

Tomatoes 94

Tossed 125

Traditional mint sauce 158

Traditional potatoes roasted with pumpkin 113

Tuna, sweet soy, lemon ginger dressing 100

Tzatziki 154

Wrap 99

Yoghurt and cucumber dip 154

A NOTE ON MEASUREMENTS

1 teaspoon = 5g ($1/6$oz)/5ml (($1/8$fl oz)

1 tablespoon = 20g ($3/4$oz)/20ml ($2/3$fl oz)

Index of Recipes

First published in 2012 by New Holland Publishers
London • Sydney • Cape Town • Auckland
www.newhollandpublishers.com • www.newholland.com.au

Garfield House 86–88 Edgware Road London W2 2EA United Kingdom
1/66 Gibbes Street Chatswood NSW 2067 Australia
Wembly Square First Floor Solan Street Gardens Cape Town 8000 South Africa
218 Lake Road Northcote Auckland New Zealand

Copyright © 2012 in text: Nicole Senior & Veronica Cuskelly
Copyright © 2012 New Holland Publishers

All rights reserved. No part of this publication may be reproduced, stored in a retrieval system or transmitted, in any form or by any means, electronic, mechanical, photocopying, recording or otherwise, without the prior written permission of the publishers and copyright holders.

A catalogue record of this book is available at the British Library

ISBN 978-1-78009-240-9

Although every effort has been made to ensure the contents of this book are accurate at the time of printing, it must not be treated as a substitute for qualified medical advice. Always consult a qualified medical practitioner. Neither the authors or the publisher can be held responsible for any loss or claim arising out of the use or misuse of the suggestions, or failure to take medical care.

Nutritional analysis used SERVE Nutrition Management System Version 5.5.006 based on the AUSNUT database.

Publisher: Fiona Schultz
Publishing manager: Lliane Clarke
Senior editor: Mary Trewby
Production manager: Olga Dementiev
Printer: Toppan Leefung Printing Ltd

10 9 8 7 6 5 4 3 2 1

Follow New Holland Publishers on
Facebook: www.facebook.com/NewHollandPublishers